Advance Praise for *Free to Be Well*©:

"I like the book so well I want to use it at my lecture series. I learned some things about nutrition I did not know. This book is packed full of information."
  Don Vradenburg, D.C., DABCI
  Mountain Lakes Chiropractic Clinic, Klamath Falls, Oregon

"As a healthcare practitioner who specializes in nutritional interventions I have been looking for useful references and methods for educating patients. Dr. Honeyman has provided up-to-date knowledge with practical lifestyle suggestions to help maintain wellness into the 50s, 60s, 70s and beyond. I commend Dr. Honeyman's efforts."
  Eleanor Barrager, A.P.D. (Accredited Practicing Dietitian)
  Genesis Center for Integrative Medicine, Graham, Washington

"I appreciated the wonderfully easy to follow explanations about body processes offered in Free to Be Well. Leaping Livers gave me several new ideas to use when talking with my patients. I want to get copies of this book into my patients' hands to help them understand more about natural approaches for wellness. It is very well put together and easily understood by professional and layperson alike. It can be the foundation to getting well."
  Virginia Hadley, RN/RC Nutritionist to Tahoma Clinic
  Medical Director Jonathon V. Wright, MD

FREE

TO BE

USING FOOD
AND SUPPLEMENTS
TO PREVENT ILLNESS

WELL

Usha Honeyman, D.C., DABCI

Published by
Dr. Oo's Publishing
975 NW Spruce Ave.
Corvallis, Oregon 97330

Library of Congress Card Number: 99-091654

Honeyman, Usha
    Free to Be Well: Using Food and Supplements to Prevent Illness

Portions of Chapter 4 adapted from *The Macrobiotic Way* by Michio Kushi and
Stephen Blauer (c) 1985, 1993. Avery Publishing Group, Inc. Garden City Park, New
York. Adapted with permission.

ISBN 0-9673767-1-8
First Edition

Cover Art and Graphics: Monica Hampton
Copy Editor: Ginnie Grilley
Illustrations: Liz Baker and Usha Honeyman

Printed by Hignell Book Printing, Winnipeg, Manitoba, Canada.

March 2000

Note to Readers:

Practicing medical freedom involves personal responsibility. This material is not intended to medically diagnose or prescribe. The author, publisher, or marketing company assume no responsibility if you diagnose or prescribe for yourself. If you have, or think you have a condition which requires medical attention, please seek qualified professional health care.

Do not change your diet if you are ill or on medication unless you are under the care of a physician. Do not change your medications without the advice of a physician.

Acknowledgments

I would like very much to thank the dedicated folks at Healthcomm International including Jeffrey Bland, Ph.D. and Eleanor Barrager, A.P.D. for their unswerving devotion to science and the education of health care providers. My thanks to the folks at Thorne Research for publishing the *Alternative Medicine Review: A Journal of Clinical Therapeutics*, a consistently excellent source of scientific information for the busy practitioner.

I would like to thank my teachers, especially those at Onondaga Community College, in Syracuse, New York. Good teachers open our minds to worlds we hadn't considered. I am lucky to have been blessed with many good teachers.

I also thank the many folks who have helped in the production of this project and were patient beyond measure through its completion. In this regard special mention must go to my friend, Ginnie Grilley for editing the manuscript.

To Paula and Kathie
for seeing this book before I considered it.

Contents

Introduction   vi

Happy Hearts   1

Giggling Guts   29

Leaping Livers   57

Demystifying Diets   87

Glad Glands   117

Danger Drugs   143

Glossary of Terms   169

Questions and Answers   176

References   179

Sources and Resources   193

Index   196

Introduction

It is my sincere hope that you will find in these pages and on the accompanying audio tapes a wealth of information and a variety of concepts that are new to you. I have tried to compile the most useful information currently available in the health sciences field to prevent disease.

We have an epidemic in the industrialized world of a terrible scourge of disease conditions. Conditions which kill thousands and thousands of people every year. These killers are heart disease, stroke, diabetes, high blood pressure, and cancer. In addition we have a Pandora's Box of debilitating diseases, which while they don't kill, usually cripple. These are diseases like arthritis, ulcerative colitis, and asthma. Despite the presence of more than ample scientific evidence that these diseases are often preventable, the necessary information to prevent these killers from striking is not getting to the public. I see folks in my practice every day who have heard that margarine is better than butter, or that a very low fat diet is good for their heart, or eliminating salt is good for their high blood pressure, or to lower their cholesterol they need to stop eating eggs and bacon. While this information is well intentioned, it barely begins to scratch the surface of what we have the power to do for our bodies in terms of keeping ourselves truly healthy.

For most of us the recommendations I will make here are a radical departure from how we currently think about health and especially from how we typically eat. I am the first to admit that I struggle to eat lots of vegetables every day and I am not always successful. But I can assure you, based on my experiences with my patients and the volumes of scientific information on diet, that if you are willing to experiment with the "kitchen" changes in *Free to Be Well*, you will reap the benefits of improved health and well being.

I undertook this project at the request of a patient because she believes I have useful information to share. I heartily agree with her, and when I took on this project, I had no idea how much work it would be. What this finished project has become is a ready source of the basic information each of my patients deserves to get. In the office, I sometimes forget to ask a person whether she eats margarine, or eats at fast food restaurants. I forget to remind one person about how important vegetables are in the diet, or the vital influence of the right type of fiber on gut function, or the importance of essential fatty acids to liver and brain health. This book and the tapes that go with it contain information that I have time to teach only in small bits for my patients. I have included a glossary of unfamiliar terms and a question and answer section after Chapter Six, which I hope will enhance your grasp of the material as you read.

As you study this material, you will find that keeping the heart healthy will also keep the liver healthy, etc. Remember the kid's game, "the ankle bone's connected to the shin bone's connected to the knee bone"? In reality everything is interrelated and the health of each of our body systems depends on the health of every other body system. The health of each of our cells has a bearing on overall health. Health is more than freedom from disease. Health means feeling wonderful. We each have a right to information that will enable us to feel vibrantly healthy and wonderful! This book is an attempt to present good, balanced information on this topic. Whether one feels well, under the weather, or has a serious disease we all have the right to information that will help us feel better and stay healthier over the long term.

Wishing you a long and happy life.

Usha Honeyman
December 1998
Corvallis, Oregon

<u>Chapter 1</u>
<u>Happy Hearts</u>

Hello and welcome to Free to Be Well©. This tape series is intended to give you useful information that will help you stay healthy over decades of life. I am Dr. Usha Honeyman and I practice as a Chiropractic Internist. I specialize in my practice in treating people who have serious diseases by using natural means. The principle treatments I prescribe to my patients are dietary modifications, nutritional supplements, and herbs. My approach to each patient is examining the functional capacity of that person's body and developing a program that maximizes their existing function and improves on any deficiencies their body may be showing.

Information I Will be Sharing With You

My goal is to give advice on these tapes that a healthy person could use to avoid illness. In other words, how do we keep our bodies healthy long term? I want to express the things I wish I could have told my patients to do long before they developed the diseases that I treat in my practice.

Common Health Advice

I would like to begin with some of the common health advice we have all heard. Here are some health topics I am sure you already know about; the importance of exercise for your heart and blood vessels, the importance of stress reduction, the importance of reducing or eliminating fats from your diet, and reducing or eliminating cholesterol in your diet. You would have had to live under a rock not to have heard discussions about low-fat, cholesterol, drinking enough water, taking vitamins and minerals, especially calcium, and don't forget, Mom said to eat your vegetables. Now, what you may not know is that these tips barely scratch the surface of the iceberg of knowledge that is available to really prevent disease.

Diets

In these tapes some of the health topics I would like to make you equally familiar with as the ones I just listed above include diets like detox diets, The Zone diet, vegan diets, macrobiotic diets, blood type diets, and hypoallergenic diets. I will also discuss nutritional supplements in detail. Briefly, these include vitamins, minerals, essential fatty acids, some amino acids, and some herbs. I will also be covering prescription and non-prescription drugs. These drugs are fraught with pitfalls for our bodies. In fact, a friend of mine who is an M.D. told me that the medical philosophy regarding drugs is that if a drug does not have serious side effects, it is not worth using because it will not do any good. Conversely, his reason for not using vitamins is that no one has ever been harmed by vitamins, therefore, they could not possibly do anything in the body.

Detoxification

I also hope to convey a thorough understanding of the topic of detoxification for today's industrial society. We need to be able to detoxify our bodies so they can heal from the effects of modern chemical, heavy metal pollution, and changes we have made in our food supply. This topic is intimately linked with cancer prevention and the normalization of immune function. I will also be covering heavy metals and their health effects. The term heavy metals encompasses things like aluminum, antimony, arsenic, beryllium, barium, cadmium, lead, mercury, silver, tin, and uranium. These minerals occur naturally in the earth, however, our bodies do not have mechanisms to get rid of them very easily. In our industrialized society we get exposed to much higher amounts of these minerals than our body can eliminate and they accumulate, causing toxic effects.

Disease Prevention

Another topic we will focus on is prevention of the leading killers including heart disease, atherosclerosis, and stroke. We will take a close look at the liver and intestines, two organs absolutely vital to our health, and how we take care of them over the long term. I'll discuss intestinal permeability, also known as leaky gut syndrome, candida or yeast overgrowth in the colon, the liver and its role in health, the overload of liver detoxification pathways, what causes this and how to help heal them. Overloaded detox liver pathways also contribute to brain poison and endocrine poison. I will discuss the endocrine system and keeping the thyroid and adrenal glands happy. In addition, we will talk about prevention of problems specific to women such as PMS and menopausal discomfort and, specific to men, prevention of prostate discomfort.

As you listen to these tapes, you will probably notice the advice for preventing many of these conditions is fairly similar from one condition to the next. Try to hear where the advice varies. The reason prevention of these conditions is similar has to do with the problems in our food supply and the all-too-common nutrient deficiencies most of us have. For example, many of us have never heard of essential fatty acids, but they are essential for a reason. Most essential fatty acids are virtually absent from our modern diets. Many diseases we see today are in part due to the absence of these nutrients in our bodies. For example, some authorities on alternative cancer treatments say that many cancers are deficiencies of certain essential fatty acids.

Heart Disease

With the introductory material out of the way, let's delve into our first in-depth topic. I chose to put prevention of heart disease and hardening of the arteries as our first topic because they are major killers in North America. Heart disease is the leading cause of death among both men and women in North America. Conditions that cause heart disease are: hardening of the arteries that bring blood to the heart muscle; heart attacks; and congestive heart failure. In addition, hardening of the arteries, or atherosclerosis, is the leading cause of stroke. Prevention of these causes is possible. On this tape, I will talk briefly about these diseases and then about natural means of preventing them.

Atherosclerosis

Atherosclerosis, or hardening of the arteries, is implicated as a causative factor in both heart attacks and stroke. Atherosclerosis starts with inflammation of the lining of the blood vessel wall. Even a tiny spot of irritation can develop and in response the body forms a blood clot. This clot adheres to the blood vessel wall. The protective clot is replaced by a tough tissue called fibrin, and bits of calcium and fats, especially the low-density cholesterol, are added. This mass is accumulating on the inside of the blood vessel wall, constantly exposed to the blood stream, and slows the blood as it flows past. This causes more cholesterol, calcium, and fibrin to fall out of the flowing blood and makes the mass continue to grow. Late in the process, a blood vessel that started as a soft, smooth, round pipe for blood to whoosh quickly through becomes almost entirely blocked by this hard, rough, growing mass of calcium, fat, and fibrin dropping out of passing blood and attaching to it. The best prevention for atherosclerosis is the prevention of the initial inflammation of the blood vessel wall. The phrase "prevention of inflammation" is important because we are going to talk about prevention of inflammation when we talk about many other topics. I am going to explain how we prevent inflammation later on this tape.

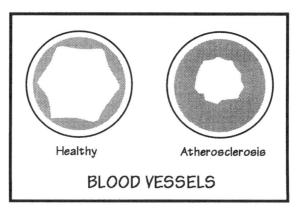

Heart Attacks

The next condition I would like to talk about is heart attack. Heart attacks are interruption of the blood supply to the heart muscle causing death to a part of that muscle. Heart attacks also cause an interruption of the heartbeat. The heart stops beating for some length of time. There is a certain threshold, of course, above which that length of time will cause death. There are two typical causes of heart attacks. Atherosclerosis of the vessels that brings blood to the heart muscles is responsible for the vast majority. The second cause of heart attacks is interruption of the heart's normal rhythm. There are a variety of things that can interrupt the heart's normal rhythm, but many rhythm disturbances are usually preventable with the right nutrients. So prevention of most heart attacks involves making sure our heart muscle has the right nutrients for correct heart rhythm and also making sure we can prevent the inflammation of the blood vessel walls that leads to atherosclerosis.

Strokes

The next condition I would like to talk about is strokes. Strokes are the interruption of the blood supply to part of the brain causing the death of some brain tissue. Things that interrupt the blood supply are usually problems with the blood vessels, and by far the major cause of stroke, again, is atherosclerosis.

Prevention!

If we can prevent that little spot of inflammation inside the blood vessel wall from starting, we can prevent some pretty tough health problems. How do we keep these blood vessel walls soft, smooth, and elastic? This is going to be a large bulk of information, so hold onto your seat!

The number one contributor to healthy blood vessels is our diet. If you think about it, the bulk of what we put in our mouths is food, not nutritional supplements. If I eat an unhealthy diet, there is no amount of nutritional supplementation or herbs I can take to make up for the damage I have done by the food I have consumed. The supplements and herbs would be totally overwhelmed by the shear volume of unhealthy foods I have put into my mouth. The number one place to start is diet. We must eat a healthy diet if we are going to get anywhere in terms of preventing diseases.

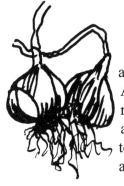

Eat Your Vegetables!

The first thing you probably expect me to talk about regarding diet and heart disease is fat. Although fat and the quality of the fats we eat are really important, the first thing I would like to talk about is vegetables. Remember, Mom always said to eat your vegetables. More and more research around the globe is showing that vegetables and fruits are rich in many kinds of nutrients that do many beneficial things in our blood stream and for our liver, brain, and heart. I implore my patients to eat a minimum of two cups per day, preferably four cups a day of non-starchy vegetables. These are vegetables like broccoli, tomatoes, cauliflower, cabbage, kale, carrots, beets, leeks, and onions. Starchy vegetables are white potato, corn, parsnip, and rutabaga. Squashes and even sweet potatoes are considered non-starchy vegetables.

The different classifications of vegetables have different types of nutrients. The brassica family (or cruciferous vegetables) which include broccoli, cauliflower, cabbage, kale, and Brussels sprouts, all have specific classes of phytonutrients. Phytonutrients are plant nutrients, many of which help in the liver detoxification pathways. Those nutrients diminish the toxic burden in the body by helping the liver eliminate toxins through normal metabolic pathways.

The yellow, orange vegetables like carrots and squashes, and red vegetables like tomatoes, have other nutrients in them, especially a broad spectrum of compounds called carotenoids. You have probably heard of beta- carotene, and more and more research has shown that we need more than just carotene or beta-carotene. We need a broad range of carotenoids. If you were shopping for a nutritional supplement, you should look for something called mixed carotenoids rather than just beta-carotene. A really easy way to get your carotenoids is to eat your yellow, orange, and red vegetables.

How You Serve Your Vegetables Matters

Before I move off the subject of vegetables, I have a pet peeve about how we eat vegetables. It is really important to eat vegetables and not drown them in fat, even if it is good quality fat. Many of my patients say they eat salad every day, and my question is, "Do you put dressing on it?" The salad dressing is one of my pet peeves. It typically has too much fat for the amount of vegetable you're eating. Another problem with salad dressing is the bottled dressings from the store or the dressings you get in a restaurant generally have oils or fats in them that are extremely poor quality and cause irritation to the liver and blood vessels.

People generally put some kind of sauce on cooked vegetables, like a hollandaise sauce or butter. I recommend people eat their vegetables steamed or lightly steamed and not add any type of fat to the vegetables at the table. This may sound like a tremendous austerity, but try it for a while and you will find that you feel better and you will learn to appreciate the taste of the vegetables. You will be able to tell whether broccoli is really fresh or not. Enough about vegetables for this tape; we'll hear more about them later.

Fats and Cholesterol in Your Diet

Let's move on to the topic I am sure you were waiting on the edge of your seat for, fats and cholesterol in the diet. Guess what? I am not going to tell you that a low-fat diet is good for your heart or blood vessels. For many folks a low-fat diet raises their bad cholesterol levels.

Let's pause here and talk briefly about cholesterol. Good cholesterol is the HDL cholesterol that stands for high-density lipo-protein. This cholesterol actually protects our cell walls and blood vessels from injury. The bad cholesterol is the LDL or low-density lipo-protein. The low-density lipo-protein or LDL cholesterol participates in that mass of "stuff" that accumulates inside vessel walls when they get inflamed causing atherosclerosis. The LDL, or bad cholesterol, tends to worsen atherosclerosis and HDL, or good cholesterol, actually helps prevent atherosclerosis. Ideally we want our HDL cholesterol to be on the higher side of normal and we want a lower LDL cholesterol level. This is to protect the blood vessels from atherosclerosis and to help prevent the complications of heart attacks and stroke.

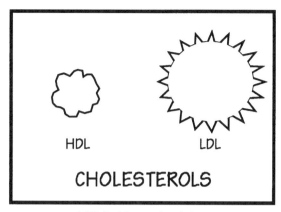

LDL is big and sticky

As I said before, very low-fat diets can raise the bad cholesterol levels. Cholesterol is made in the liver from starches, sugars, and carbohydrates that we consume. We get some cholesterol in our blood stream from our diet, but 80% of total cholesterol circulating in the blood is not from the cholesterol in our diet. It is made by the liver from the carbohydrates or starches that we eat. If the liver lacks good-quality fats and lacks any vitamins or minerals that it needs for normal processes, then it cannot properly handle starches. Cholesterol levels will rise in the blood because the liver is making too much LDL cholesterol.

An especially detrimental version of the low-fat diets is the diet that is based mainly on starches that are refined, like white pastas and white bread. These refined starches are devoid of the spectrum of minerals and B-vitamins that occur naturally in the whole grain kernel. These refined starches actually force the liver to divert vitamins and minerals from other things that the liver is trying to do.

You may wonder why I am talking so much about the liver. One of the things that is known about the liver is that nobody has discovered how many chemical reactions it participates in within our bodies. We will talk about the liver more on another tapc. It suffices to say that what is going on in the liver has a direct bearing on the health of our blood vessels and the amount of inflammation happening in the blood stream and against the blood vessel walls.

Fats are Necessary for a Healthy Body

Believe it or not, studies are showing that people need good quality fats, including essential fatty acids, in order to help keep cholesterol levels low. In fact, some cultures in the world that have relatively high-fat diets have fairly low rates of heart disease. This is exemplified by some of the Mediterranean cultures where olive oil is a high percentage of the diet, and the Scandinavian, far North American Eskimos, and Inuit peoples who eat a high percentage of fat in their diet but have very low rates of heart disease when they eat their indigenous diets.

Good Fats

The "take home" to remember regarding fats is that fats in the diet can be either good fats or bad fats. Good fats include fish oils and some of the monounsaturated oils; olive oil is a beneficial fat for many reasons. The term "fat" means oils and lipids generally. I hope I haven't confused you. From the health care perspective, fats are fats. Whether they are in an oil form or a solid fat form, they are all fats to us. The beneficial fish oils are the oils in "fins and scales" type fish. These are fish like halibut, sardines, and salmon. Shellfish do not have the beneficial oils in them. Shellfish are seafood like crab, shrimp, clams, oysters, etc.

Vegetable oils can be either monounsaturated or polyunsaturated. Many of us have been taught that polyunsaturated oils are the best oils to use. The truth is that monounsaturated vegetable oils are the healthiest forms of oils for cooking and eating. Monounsaturated oils are principally canola and olive oil. Remember, Mediterranean cultures in which people eat a lot of olive oil have been shown to have low levels of heart disease and hardening of the arteries. Olive oil is number one on the list of good fats for people to eat on a regular basis. Another very excellent fat to consume in the diet is flaxseed oil. Flaxseed is rich in the omega 3 essential fatty acids that help to lower cholesterol and prevent inflammation on a cellular level. Fatty acids in flaxseed are subject to rapid deterioration, so once they are ground, they need to be eaten quickly. They should be kept in Mother Nature's container (that is the seed) until shortly before you're going to eat them.

The reason olive oil is number one on my list is because of ease of use. You can go to the supermarket and buy a bottle of oil for whatever you chose to in your kitchen. The oil in flaxseed is actually healthier than olive oil, but is harder to come by. If you want to purchase flaxseed oil already extracted from the seed, you need to be extremely careful about the product you buy. The oil should be extracted from the seed at low temperatures so it does not get heated and turn rancid. Once it has been extracted from the seed, the oil needs to be kept refrigerated until you actually consume it. Alternately, some flaxseed oil products are available now where the oil is either in liquid form or capsule form and has been preserved by natural means to protect it against oxidation or rancidification. In very few products the oil can be at room temperature and the essential fatty acids, or omega 3 fatty acids, are preserved in the flax oil. The best way to know that you are getting the essential fatty acids from flax is to keep the seeds in your house and grind them just before you are going to eat them. Flax seeds are cheap and easy to grind with an electric grinder such as a spice or coffee grinder. The dose to take per day is between 1 and 3 tablespoons. It has a pleasant flavor similar to walnuts. You can sprinkle them on your food. If you cook with the ground seed, it will destroy the essential fatty acids, so keep it at room temperature or refrigerated until you eat it.

Another excellent source of essential fatty acids is in supplements. You can find these oils in capsules in the health food stores. Evening primrose oil and black currant oil are rich in some of the essential fatty acids that are hard to get in our diets. We will discuss these later under nutritional supplements. Recall, it's very difficult to come by essential fatty acids in the modern diet. If our food supply was completely natural, we would be getting essential fatty acids from whole grains kept in kernel form until they are ground into flour to cook the same day or same week and from fresh nuts which are high in essential fatty acids. For most of us, the foods we eat are processed sometimes years before we actually consume them. The essential fatty acids are either absent or have gone rancid; the fats in these foods can actually do us more harm than good.

Bad Fats

So what about our promised list of bad fats? Bad fats include: polyunsaturated vegetable oils, hydrogenated fats, margarine, cottonseed oils, and animal fats. I will explain each of these in more detail. First, polyunsaturated versus saturated fats, with an explanation about the fat molecule.

Fat molecules are long chains of carbon atoms with hydrogen atoms attached to them. Saturated fats have all available carbon bonds filled with hydrogen atoms. So, on the long chain of carbon atoms in a saturated fat, every single available bond on the carbons is attached to an hydrogen. A monounsaturated fat is again a long chain of atoms with one available bond; all the available bonds on the carbon atoms are filled with hydrogens except for one bond on each chain of the fat. This makes it monounsaturated (mono being one). A polyunsaturated fat or oil has many available bonds to attach things to. In this long chain of

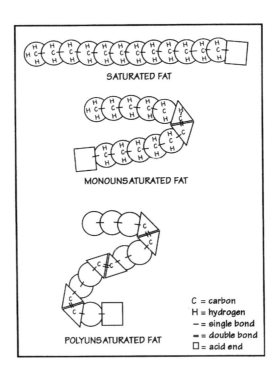

carbon atoms there are a lot of available double bonds between the carbons that can attach to things like hydrogen. A polyunsaturated fat tends to be liquid at room temperature and a saturated fat will tend to be more solid at room temperature. The saturated fat molecule is the most stable, least likely to go rancid or oxidize. If you don't know what oxidation is, rust is an example of oxidation of iron. Oxidation occurs when oxygen reacts with things and causes damage. You've probably heard of nutritional supplements that are anti-oxidants. These are a whole class of supplements that protect our cells from the damage that oxygen can cause them.

Manufacturing Bad Fats

Chemically altered fats such as margarine fall in the category of hydrogenated fats. Margarine damages blood vessel walls, raises the LDL (bad cholesterol levels), tends to lower the HDL level (good cholesterol levels), and increases the inflammatory and allergic reactions in the blood stream. Margarine is a cause of atherosclerosis, the inflammation and hardening of blood vessel walls. Hydrogenated fats start as polyunsaturated vegetable oils. They are liquid at room temperature and have lots of available carbon bonds. These vegetable oils are brought to extremely high temperatures while hydrogen is bubbled through them to hydrogenate them. The hydrogen attaches to the available, highly reactive double bonds and opens them up. This changes these fats from polyunsaturated to fully saturated with hydrogen. Saturation allows margarine to stay solid like butter at room temperature.

If you put the pieces together about the differences between monounsaturated, saturated, and polyunsaturated fats, you understand when we hydrogenate an oil we turn it from a polyunsaturated to a fully saturated oil. Through a chemical process we have created a fully saturated fat. It is beyond me why scientists believe that an artificially saturated fat is better for us than a naturally saturated fat. In fact, the statistics in this country about hardening of the arteries, stroke, and heart disease do not bear out that the inclusion of margarine and hydrogenated fats in our diet has been a good thing over the decades that they have been part of our diet.

I hope I didn't bore you with this biochemistry. I want you to understand margarine and other hydrogenated fats are very unhealthy for us. Remember, hydrogenated fats damage blood vessel walls and cell walls, raise the LDL, lower the HDL, increase inflammatory reactions, and increase allergic reactions in the blood stream that damage our cells. When you're shopping in the supermarket and are reading labels, please read the fine print on the foods you buy to take home to your kitchen. Foods that are most likely (and this is not a complete list) to have hydrogenated oils and fats in them are: margarine, baked goods such as prepared cookies, cakes, canned icing, cake mixes, pancake mixes, and crackers.

Peanut butter is another major source of hydrogenated oils. If you like peanut butter, experiment with the natural peanut butters that don't contain hydrogenated oils. It may take some getting used to their flavors, but, in the long run, you will notice that they actually taste more like peanuts. These peanut butters are peanuts and salt; they don't have the damaging hydrogenated oils in them.

Not Meant for Human Consumption

The next bad-for-you fat is cottonseed oil. Cotton, as we all know, is not grown for food. Therefore, many farm chemicals, toxic pesticides and herbicides and other chemicals are used on a cotton crop that are not allowed on food crops. When the cottonseed is extracted from the cotton and oil is extracted from the seed, it has the residues of toxic chemicals in it. These residues make cottonseed oil a very unhealthy oil to consume. When you are looking at any fried snack food, suspect cottonseed oil, especially in potato chips, corn chips, etc. Read ingredients! Please avoid cottonseed oil in your diet.

Animal Fats

The next subject regarding fat, is animal fat. In general animal fats are not good to consume. One exception is butter or clarified butter (also known as ghee.) The reason for this exception is for folks who want margarine or butter on their food. I much prefer butter to margarine for all the reasons listed above regarding problems caused by hydrogenated oils.

Sources of animal fats include: red meats (like beef and pork), poultry (like chicken and turkey), fish, and dairy products. Dairy products include milk, cream, half-and-half, butter, cheese, yogurt, and ice cream. There are a wide variety of cheeses with a wide variety of fat contents. The main reason animal fat is a problem is that most of us eat such a high percentage of animal foods in the North American diet. Animal fats have an essential fatty acid called arachidonic acid which we *do* need. However, we tend to eat an imbalance of essential fatty acids. Most of us get much more arachidonic acid than we need and we don't get the other essential fatty acids for reasons I explained previously. When we consume too much arachidonic acid and not enough other essential fatty acids, it pushes the inflammatory reaction in our body to accelerate. This causes us more pain or inflammation generally. Specifically, it gives impetus to that little spot of inflammation starting the atherosclerotic process on the wall of the vein or artery.

In the North American diet, we eat larger portions of animal protein foods which also contain more fat than our body really needs. Regarding portions, I recommend people keep their animal protein portions, poultry and red meats, to a 4 oz. size. That is about the size of the palm of your hand. None of these 14 and 16 oz. steaks! They're not good for you. You also should keep dairy products to 4 oz. servings. Larger servings of high protein foods are very hard on the body for a number of reasons. Not just because of the fat, but also because of the high protein and the chemicals that come along with commercially raised animal products.

One way to get a much better quality fat in our diet is to eat only meats and poultry that are free range or grass fed. Animals have a unique feature that the cell membranes in our bodies are made of the fats that we eat in our diet, so the type of fats that we eat will then translate into what type of fats our cells use to make cell membranes. This has a direct bearing on health, the immune system, and disease processes generally. In other words, healthy cell membranes and good quality fats in our cell membranes will help keep our immune system from over-reacting. Good quality fats help diminish allergic reactions and metabolic inflammation in the body. One way to get these good essential fatty acids and avoid the inflammatory essential fatty acids is to eat animals fed green foods. Grass-fed beef, free-range poultry, and wild salmon have fat in their tissues that is rich in omega 3 essential fatty acids. Omega 3 essential fatty acids are actually anti-inflammatory. Corn fed meats and fish that are fed corn (in other words farm fish) are high in fats that cause inflammation.

This doesn't mean it's OK to eat a lot of meat, because a high meat diet is not healthy for your heart or your liver. What it means is that if we're going to eat meats and poultry, we should get the free-range poultry and grass-fed beef. Keep the portion sizes on your poultry, meats, fishes, and dairy products to 4 oz. per meal.

How Much Fat Is Healthy

The last topic I would like to cover on fat is the amount of fats to eat. Figure this as a percentage of your total calories per day. No matter how many calories you eat in a day, you should have 30% or less of those calories as fat. Some diets allow far less than 30% of the total calories as fat; we will talk about different types of diets on Tape Four. Thirty percent is the maximum fat calories you should be taking in. If you're like me and don't know how to count calories, I'll give you some helpful hints.

The foods we eat are all made of protein, carbohydrate (also known as starch), and fat. The fats are very calorie-dense foods. For one tablespoon of food, if it is protein or starch, it has an equal amount of calories. If that tablespoon is a tablespoon of fat or oils, it has double the calories, roughly, of a tablespoon of any other food. In order to keep the total volume of fat in the diet below one-third or roughly 30% calories, you have to keep the volume of fat or oil in the diet below one-sixth of the total volume of food you eat. For every six tablespoons of food you are eating, fat should be no more than one tablespoon. Some diets we will talk about on Tape Four will allow a maximum of 1-2 tablespoons of fat per day.

Remember also that when you are eating foods, if they are cooked in oil, they absorb the oil, so think of that in terms of the volume of fat you are getting. Watch for those hidden fats in foods, for example spaghetti sauce in a jar often has a lot of oil in it and we don't necessarily think of that as a fatty food.

Fiber and Its Effect on Heart Disease

The next topic we'll cover is fiber and its effect on heart disease. An important aspect about fiber is that not all fibers are created equal. What is fiber? Fiber is contained in vegetable foods, grains, beans, fruits, and vegetables. It is not digestible and does not provide any calories or nutrition for us. However, fiber is extremely important for our health. Most of us think of fiber as something that helps us have regular bowel movements by bulking up our stools. This is only the tip of the iceberg regarding the vital role fiber plays in the diet. We are going to talk about the things fiber can do for us on Tape Two, but just remember not all fibers are created equal.

Just as you might chose clothing of cotton or silk because of the properties of the fiber and how it feels, fibers in our diet are not generic. Fiber in food is either soluble or insoluble. Pectin, in many fruits, is a soluble fiber. Soluble fiber in the diet is very important for lowering cholesterol. Soluble fiber aids in lowering cholesterol by binding with cholesterol in the intestines and carrying it out of the body in our stools. In the absence of soluble fiber, cholesterol gets re-absorbed from the colon into the blood stream, keeping the cholesterol level in our blood high. Sources of soluble fiber include fruits and vegetables, especially apples. Whole grains and beans, soy, flaxseed, garlic, and onions are all good sources of soluble fiber. Insoluble fibers are those like wheat bran.

One of my pet peeves are the instructions to take a fiber supplement daily to aid with bowel movements. Many of the products you buy in the drug store are mainly insoluble fiber. They may contain wheat bran which can be extremely irritating to the mucosal lining of the colon. In contrast, there are some types of fiber which promote the growth of beneficial species of bacteria in the colon. This enhances the environment in the colon and a normal ecosystem in the colon is vitally important for overall health. We will talk about colon health on Tape Two.

Carbohydrates

The next subject we'll discuss regarding diet and health of the heart and blood vessels is carbohydrates. Carbohydrates are in our diet in the form of sugars and in the form of starches. We have all been told since we were little that sugar isn't healthy. Refined sugars are very hard on the body for a variety of reasons. Mainly because refined sugars deplete minerals like magnesium and several B vitamins when our liver tries to metabolize them. Refined sugar is in our diet principally in the form of white sugar. Candies, cookies, cakes, pastries, desserts, etc. all use refined sugar. These foods should be kept to a minimum in our diet in order to avoid disease in general and especially to avoid disease of the arteries and the heart.

Starches are present in our diet mainly from grains and also from starchy vegetables such as potatoes or corn. When grains are refined, they lose minerals and vitamins. The same thing happens when we eat white flour that happens when we eat white sugar. Our body gets depleted of B vitamins and certain minerals in order for us to digest the white flour products. White flour is used in bread, cookies, bagels, pastries, etc. In the standard North American diet we must go out of our way to get breads, cakes, and cookies made from whole grain flours. However, in order to get a full compliment of vitamins and minerals with our grains, the whole grain needs to be present in the food. The best way to envision this is to think about fixing food from scratch and starting with the whole-wheat kernel. The wheat kernel has the wheat germ which is most of the protein, it has the starchy part around the wheat germ, and then it has the husk or bran. All of those components need to be present when you eat wheat in order to get a full compliment of vitamins, minerals, and proteins that Mother Nature packaged in the wheat kernel.

Summary of Dietary Recommendations

To summarize my dietary recommendations for prevention of atherosclerosis and heart disease. First, I ask people to eat lots and lots of vegetables. Second, I ask that you eliminate the bad fat from your diet and include good quality fats in moderation. Third, don't eat very much protein. If you are going to eat meat products, keep the portions to 4 oz. or less. Fourth, include fiber in your diet in the foods you eat rather than as an over-the-counter type fiber supplement. Last, have your carbohydrates as whole grains and beans and not as refined sugars and white flour products. Remember, pastas are carbohydrates and are available as whole grain dishes. People forget pasta is made from grain and most pasta in the supermarket is universally a white flour product. You can find whole grain pastas in health food stores, food coops, and other similar shops.

Where to Shop

This brings me to a very good point. You're probably thinking, "Where am I going to get these foods this nutty person is telling me to eat?" In the United States, you generally have to go out of your way to find these foods, but they *are* available in most communities. The place to try is a health food store or an alternative type food coop. In some communities there are even alternative grocery stores as large as most supermarkets. These alternative grocery stores are filled with organically raised meats, free-range chicken, whole grain pasta, and whole grain breads, etc. The first time you go in one of those stores, leave yourself a lot of time to read ingredients and discover their variety of products.

Exercise

When we talk about the prevention of heart disease, a topic certainly not to be neglected is exercise. Regular aerobic exercise, at least 20-25 minutes of exercise per day at least 3-4 days per week is vitally important for the health of the heart and blood vessels. Exercise can be as simple as going for a walk or walking your dog 20 minutes three days a week. It does not have to be anything elaborate or expensive, just something that gets your heart pumping and gets the blood moving through your vessels.

Nutritional Supplements

Our next topic is nutritional supplements and prevention of heart disease and atherosclerosis. Keep in mind throughout this whole discussion of nutritional supplements, the biggest volume of stuff we put in our mouths is our diet, the foods we eat. No amount of nutritional supplements you can take will make up for a diet filled with junk food. Therefore, you must consider diet as the first priority among these nutritional recommendations.

I have divided these supplements arbitrarily into four groups, but there is quite a bit of overlap among them. The first group are those that lower cholesterol, the second group are those that dissolve plaquing, third are supplements that improve heart muscle function, and fourth are supplements improving circulation. Some of these supplements are vitamins, some are minerals, some are enzymes, and some are herbs.

Supplements that Lower Cholesterol

Among supplements that lower cholesterol, the two most easily available and very effective supplements are niacin and garlic. Both niacin and garlic work better at lowering total cholesterol than prescription drugs. Niacin and garlic also lower total triglycerides, which are fats in the blood, and they raise HDL cholesterol (good cholesterol). This means these natural agents actually do a better job of managing and maintaining optimal fat content in the blood. They keep the total cholesterol low, bring up the good cholesterol, and bring down the triglycerides.

Interestingly, if your cholesterol is too low, niacin will also bring it up. My patients give me funny looks when I tell them their cholesterol is too low. Cholesterol is very important for many functions in the body, and our bodies make cholesterol from the carbohydrates we eat. In fact, 80% of the cholesterol circulating in our blood stream is made by the liver from carbohydrates or starches that we eat and does not come from dietary cholesterol. The reason the liver makes cholesterol is because it is vital for so many functions in our body. Cholesterol is the building block for many of the hormones made by our endocrine glands.

Niacin

Niacin should be taken in the form of inositol hexaniacinate. This is a form of niacin with six niacin molecules bound to one molecule of inositol (another B vitamin). Inositol hexaniacinate makes the niacin get released gradually over time. Otherwise plain niacin causes a flushing reaction that many people find extremely uncomfortable. This inositol hexaniacinate is not the same as timed release niacin. The chemical name of timed-release niacin is niacinamide. Niacinamide can cause temporary inflammation of the liver in a small percentage of people. Hence, most clinicians have gone to recommending inositol hexaniacinate for people who want to take niacin. There is no problem with taking the regular niacin, plain old vitamin B3, as long as you do not mind the flushing. During the flushing reaction folks get really hot and red and their skin gets itchy all over. Some people, as I said, find this extremely uncomfortable.

Niacin Dosage

The dosage of niacin for keeping cholesterol low is 500 mg 2-3 times daily. Many people find niacin gives them an energy boost and that they feel more comfortable when they take it. If you try niacin and like it, you can take up to 3000 mg or 3 gm per day with meals.

Please note, I will not talk on these tapes about specific treatment for disease. The information provided in Free to Be Well© is intended to help people stay well. However, if you have gout, the uric acid in your blood runs high, or you have diabetes, you should not take high doses of niacin. For these three groups of people, folks with high uric acid, folks with gout, and people with diabetes, keep your niacin intake below 500 mg per day.

A brief introduction to the units on nutritional supplements is called for here. Things are either labeled with milligrams (mg), micrograms (mcg), or grams (gm). Some supplements are labeled with international units which is "IU". Grams, milligrams, and micrograms differ by a factor of 1000. There are 1000 micrograms (mcg) in a milligram (mg), and there are 1000 milligrams (mg) in a gram (gm). So, 3 gm per day of niacin or hexiniacinate, is the same as taking 3000 mg per day. I'll let you figure out how many micrograms that is. My math isn't quite that good.

Garlic

Garlic is also very effective at lowering cholesterol and raising the HDL cholesterol. The dose of garlic, if you like eating fresh raw garlic, is one to two cloves per day. If you don't like either the taste or odor of garlic and want a preparation that will give you the same benefits as garlic, there are many available as nutritional supplements. You want a total allicin (the active enzyme in garlic) potential of 4000 mcg per day.

Pantethine

Another supplement that has been shown to lower cholesterol is pantethine. This is an active form of vitamin B5. Vitamin B5 is called pantothenic acid. Pantethine inhibits cholesterol synthesis and increases our body's utilization of fat as an energy source. Like niacin and garlic, pantethine lowers total cholesterol, lowers triglycerides, and raises HDL or good cholesterol. Dosage on pantethine should be between 300 mg and 900 mg per day.

If you are concerned about keeping your cholesterol low and want to take any of these supplements, there is no need to do all three. My suggestion is to pick one, either niacin, garlic, or pantethine, try it, and see how your cholesterol does.

Supplements that Dissolve Plaquing

The next category of supplements are things that dissolve plaques. I will also include things that help prevent plaque from forming. Supplements that help prevent plaque are generally enzymes. If you have a severe case of atherosclerosis, this is by no means a treatment, so please don't consider it such. This information is intended to help folks stay healthy and to help prevent plaquing from forming on blood vessel walls. These supplements also prevent inflammation.

This group of supplements is almost exclusively digestive enzymes, especially enzymes that help digest protein. In order to have an anti-inflammatory effect (remember anything that is anti-inflammatory will help protect blood vessel walls), enzymes should be taken between meals rather than with food. One of the best enzymes that digests protein is bromelain. This enzyme is derived from the stems of pineapple. It is highly concentrated pineapple. If you have an allergy to pineapple, please do not use bromelain.

Dosages of enzymes vary from product to product because the potency of the capsule or tablet is based on the activity level or strength of the enzyme each manufacturer uses. With a reasonably good quality product, I have people take from two to six tablets daily. For folks with an allergy to pineapple, the next best thing is a vegetable based digestive enzyme with protease in it. Protease enzymes help digest protein. The dosage is the same as it is for the bromelain, from two to six capsules daily.

Supplements that help prevent plaque are things that help prevent inflammation. Nutrients most people are deficient in that prevent inflammation are essential fatty acids, especially omega 3 and omega 6. The best way to supplement these is with flaxseed oil, borage oil, evening primrose oil, black currant oil, or fish oil. These can be found in capsule form. Flaxseed oil is also available in a liquid form. I have patients take from two to six capsules daily or a tablespoon of liquid oil. Essential fatty acids, again, help minimize inflammation in the body, help minimize allergic reactions, and generally calm down immune system reactivity that initiates irritation on the blood vessel walls.

Part of what damages blood vessel walls is oxidation of the LDL (bad cholesterol) and irritation that happens because of the LDL oxidation. There are two other classes of supplements that help prevent oxidation. One class is antioxidants. Antioxidant supplements are beta-carotene (also available in mixed carotenoids), vitamin C, vitamin E, lipoic acid, and selenium, among many others. You can take from 25,000 to 100,000 IU of beta-carotene per day. If your skin starts turning orange, you should take less beta-carotene. I try to get people to take at least 1000 mg of vitamin C per day. Between 1000 and 3000 mg per day is a healthy dose of vitamin C. With vitamin E, I try to get people to take at least 400 IU. Many good quality multi-vitamin, multi-mineral products will provide that much vitamin E. Lipoic acid, which you may not have heard of previously, is an excellent antioxidant that helps recycle vitamin C, vitamin E, and beta-carotene back to their useful forms once they have done their antioxidant thing. Lipoic acid turns them back into their original forms. Lipoic acid is also an excellent antioxidant in its own right. I recommend folks take it with food at doses between 100 mg and 600 mg per day. (A caution regarding lipoic acid: it may lower blood sugar quickly in some folks, please take it with food.) Selenium is a mineral and an excellent antioxidant. It should be taken in doses of about 100 mcg per day. Again, a good quality multi-vitamin, multi-mineral should contain 100 mcg of Selenium.

The next class of vitamins that prevent plaques are B vitamins associated with methionine and homocysteine metabolism. You may have heard recently about the discovery that increased levels of homocysteine in the blood predispose people to heart disease. This is because homocysteine increases oxidation of the bad cholesterol, aggravating the blood vessel walls and causing atherosclerosis. The way to prevent the build up of homocysteine and protect against oxidation is by making sure you are getting plenty of folic acid, B12, and B6 in your diet or by supplementation. A minimum dose of folic acid and B12 is 400 mcg of each. I try to get people to double that, and you can safely take 1200 mcg of each. Folic acid and B12 are nontoxic. Vitamin B6 dosages range from a minimum of 10 mg per day up to 50 mg per day is fine. A good quality multi-vitamin, multi-mineral product should have all of the antioxidants and B vitamins I just listed in adequate doses except lipoic acid which will not be present in sufficient doses.

I tell my patients if you are healthy and you take a good quality multi-vitamin, multi-mineral product regularly, you get what you need in terms of supplementation to keep you healthy. So if you are already healthy and want to protect your liver, heart, and blood vessels from the wear and tear of life, eat a good diet, exercise, and take a good quality multi-vitamin, multi-mineral. You do not need to go out of your way to get other supplements.

Supplements that Improve Heart Muscle Function

The principle supplement that improves heart muscle function and has been studied quite a bit is the enzyme CoQ-10. This is an enzyme used in all of our cells. We have energy factories in our cells called mitochondria. Mitochondria make the energy currency our cells use to do the things they need to do. Whether it is a muscle cell lifting hundreds of pounds of weight, or an intestinal cell doing its thing absorbing food, all of our cells need mitochondria to make energy for them. CoQ-10 is used inside the mitochondria for energy manufacture and is essential. Our bodies can make CoQ-10, but to help prevent heart muscle problems, CoQ-10 has been shown to be an important supplement. The dosage of CoQ-10 can vary widely from one person to another, so I generally start people at a low dosage and work up.

Taurine is an amino acid that helps improve heart muscle function. The usual dosage of taurine is between 500 and 2000 mg per day. L-carnitine is an amino acid that also helps heart muscle function. I generally have people start with about 300 mg per day of L-carnitine. Vitamin E helps improve heart muscle function and, again, the dose is a minimum of 400 IU per day.

Supplements that Improve Circulation

The best known supplement that improves circulation is gingko. However, any bioflavonoids will improve circulation. Pycnogenol compounds will also improve circulation. Regarding pycnogenol compounds, there are many, many plants that have pycnogenols in them. One of the highest sources of pycnogenols are grapes that have any reddish tint. Concord grapes and red flame grapes are high in pycnogenols. The herb hawthorne also helps to improve circulation, especially to the heart muscle. The dosages of herbs are anywhere from 1-4 capsules per day.

Other than precautions I've already made previously, none of these supplements should cause any problems to healthy individuals. However, if you try any supplement and you don't feel well or have any type of adverse reaction, the supplement is probably causing it, and you should discontinue it. A note about CoQ-10, I have seen patients who take it and it improves their energy level so much they have become more energetic than they preferred. If you tend to be on the high-strung side, I would not recommend CoQ-10.

With that I have come to the end of my material on heart disease and hardening of the arteries. I hope this tape has been interesting, and I hope you enjoy Tape Two.

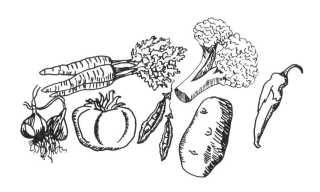

Chapter 2
Giggling Guts

Hi, and welcome to the second tape of the Free to Be Well© series. On Tape Two we are going to talk about intestinal permeability, the hidden culprit. You may not have heard of intestinal permeability, but I hope to explain it well here. Intestinal permeability is also known as leaky gut syndrome. There are many health problems associated with this condition, and they tend to be chronic and debilitating. Health problems linked to intestinal permeability include: candida infections or yeast infections, inflammatory arthritis, chronic fatigue syndrome, asthma, dermatitis, inflammatory bowel disease, intestinal malabsorption, alcoholism, and food sensitivities.

The Gastrointestinal System

In order to explain how intestinal permeability happens, we need to review the basic gastrointestinal (or digestive system) functions. The purpose of our digestive system is to provide our body calories by digesting and absorbing our food. We take in things from outside our body and process them in such a way that our cells are able to use the resulting compounds for making energy. The digestive tract is a continuous tube from our mouth to the other end. Technically the inside of this tube is really outside our body. In other words, things from

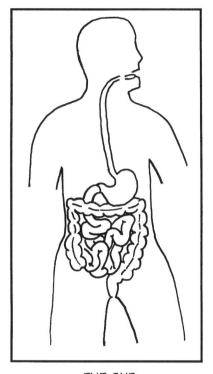

THE GUT

outside our body go into this tube, and our blood stream and visceral organs need to be protected from whatever we might ingest along with the food we are intending to eat. We generally consume a variety of microorganisms and other toxic things when we eat our food. Part of the purpose of the digestive tract is to protect us from toxic things eaten with our food. These are kept from our blood stream, while at the same time, the digestive tract absorbs nutrients into the blood stream.

The Mouth

Digestion has a variety of events that happen, one after the other. The first thing that happens when we eat is we put food in our mouths. There is an enzyme in the mouth called salivary amylase that starts digesting starches in the food. Digestion actually starts when we chew. Chewing food well is important so the foods get mixed well with the enzyme in our saliva.

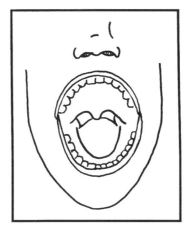

DIGESTION STARTS HERE!

The Stomach

Once we swallow the food, it goes to the stomach where stomach acid and pepsin start breaking down proteins in the food. The breakdown of protein begins in the stomach and continues in the small intestines. Food generally spends between 30 and 60 minutes in the stomach. The heavier the meal you eat or the more protein, the more time the food will spend in your stomach. The less protein you eat in the meal, the quicker the food will exit the stomach.

Many of us are used to worrying about having too much stomach acid, but a far more common problem I see clinically is people with too little stomach acid. Once we get over above age 40 to 45, the stomach cells making the acid decrease. This results in less acid in the stomach and causes insufficient breakdown of proteins in the stomach. The decrease in stomach acid doesn't impact only our digestion. It decreases the absorption of vitamins, especially B12. The decrease in absorption of B12 from the stomach as stomach acid drops will cause a decrease in activity of other B vitamins. B vitamin deficiency will worsen

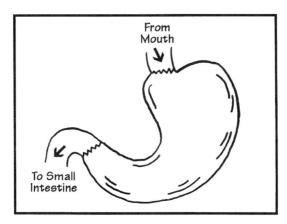

STOMACH STARTS PROTEIN DIGESTION

proportionately to the loss of stomach acid. The decrease in B vitamins will further contribute to a drop in GI (gastrointestinal) function.

To summarize digestion thus far, the normal function of the stomach is the beginning of the breakdown of proteins in food. Starch digestion starts in the mouth and protein digestion starts in the stomach.

The Small Intestines

The next step in digestion takes place in the small intestines. The stomach is a muscular bag that squirts bits of food out into the small intestine. When food mixed with stomach acid arrives in the small intestine, the pancreas is stimulated to release enzymes into the small intestines that start breaking down fats and continue breaking down the starches and proteins in the foods. The more stomach acid that arrives in the small intestine, the more digestive enzymes the pancreas will produce.

When stomach acid decreases, we will also have less breakdown by pancreatic enzymes of the molecules we consume when we eat. Starches, proteins, and fats don't get broken down as well because there aren't enough pancreatic enzymes to adequately mix with the food. Remember that the ultimate purpose of digestion is to break the starches, proteins, and fats that we eat into small enough usable units for our liver and the cells of our body to use as building blocks or to make energy. When digestion by pancreatic enzymes decreases, we will have a corresponding decrease in absorption of nutrients from the intestines into the blood stream.

If you took the whole GI tract and laid it out flat and took all the folds and bends out of it, it would have a surface area equal to a tennis court. The main purpose of that surface area is to absorb things that we eat into the blood stream. If starches, proteins and fats don't get broken down properly by enzymes, then absorption becomes much more difficult.

The Gall Bladder and Bile

Let's continue to follow the food on its journey. Near where the pancreatic enzymes get excreted into the intestines, the bile also follows hard on its heels. Bile is made in the liver, and is concentrated in the gall bladder. Bile is excreted into the small intestine just past the stomach with the pancreatic enzymes. Bile acts like a detergent, by

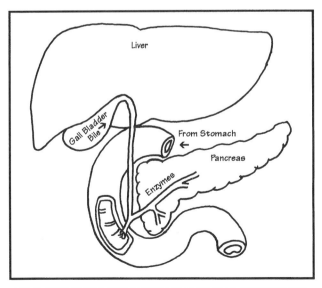

BILE AND ENZYMES ENTER THE SMALL INTESTINES FOR DIGESTION

emulsifying fats in our food so the water soluble pancreatic enzymes can digest them. Another purpose of bile is for the liver to get rid of things that do not belong in the blood stream. The liver also excretes some of its waste products in bile so that those things can go out in the stool.

Breaking our Food Down

So far we have discussed: saliva which digests starch; stomach acid that starts protein breakdown; enzymes from the pancreas which digest protein, starch, and fat; and bile in the gall bladder to help break down fat. The next process in the intestines is the continual mixing and churning with these chemicals made by our bodies that break down the food. The whole huge surface of the mucosal lining of the intestines absorbs these nutrients into the blood stream. Hopefully, we have broken them down thoroughly before we absorb them.

Hormones

In addition to the enzymes, stomach acid, and bile, there is an intricate interplay of a variety of hormones made in the stomach and small intestines that are essential for normal digestion. Some of these hormones are prostaglandins.

Our body also makes prostaglandins that are released during inflammation. These prostaglandins cause pain. Many times when people have pain (joint pain, headaches, or muscle pain), they take ibuprofen. Ibuprofen inhibits all prostaglandin synthesis. By inhibiting prostaglandin synthesis generally in the body, ibuprofen interferes with digestion. The prostaglandin hormones made in the stomach and small intestine are very important for digestion. Ibuprofen and other non-steroidal anti-inflammatories inhibit the ability of the stomach and small intestines to make their prostaglandins, and therefore these drugs interfere with proper digestion. This is the mechanism by which ibuprofen and similar non-steroidal anti-inflammatories will give people a stomachache. The drug directly interferes with the function of the stomach and small intestines.

The Large Intestine

Moving from the small intestine (which is primarily responsible for digestion and absorption), we go on to the large intestine. The large intestine is much more than a place to absorb back the liquids from the small intestines into the blood stream before the stool goes into the toilet. The large intestine, or colon, has a complex ecosystem that has an intricate interplay with the rest of our body. It is very important for the environment of the colon to be healthy. Like any other ecosystem we are familiar with (like oceans, forests, streams, etc.) that require a full range of plant and animal life to be healthy, our colon, or large intestine, requires a full range of species or organisms in a delicate balance with each other in a healthy soil. The soil in this ecosystem is the mucous membrane that lines the colon. The environment in the colon won't be healthy if what feeds it (the stomach and small intestine) aren't healthy and working properly.

Our immune system and liver are dependent on a healthy environment in the colon for us to be healthy. The immune system and liver are very important. I hope this hints at how important the large intestine's health is to the rest of our body. Well over fifty percent of our immune system is located in the GI tract. The majority of this is in the small and large intestines. There are many antibodies made by the mucosal membranes, lymph nodes, and white blood cells located inside the gut or the digestive tract. The immune system in the gut is there to protect our blood stream from organisms that we might ingest.

When the gut ecosystem and the immune system in the gut are in balance with each other, white blood cells and antibodies in the gut are able to attack and destroy invading organisms before they enter the blood stream and before they damage the mucosal lining of the digestive tract. In order for the immune system to do a good job of destroying invaders, it needs the cooperation and help of the organisms that live in the colon. Normally there are about four hundred different species of bacteria living on the mucosal surface of the large intestine. There are more organisms in each tablespoon of stool than all the stars that have ever been counted in the sky. These four hundred species have a relationship with each other. The beneficial species should be the vast majority of bacteria that live on the mucosa. There are normally bad species present, but those should be a small minority of the total organisms present.

Good Bacteria

Before you get totally grossed out about all the bacteria normally present in our gut, pause to hear what they do. In a healthy gut the good species should be the vast majority of those colonizing the mucosa. They cover the delicate mucosal lining of the colon and make several compounds that are actively anti-microbial. This means normally we have a huge number of organisms in the colon making compounds that help our bodies fight infections. These bacteria make natural antibiotic substances and protect us from infections, not just infections in the colon, but infections in the blood stream as well. The good bacteria lining the colon make vitamins that are absorbed into the blood stream. This is the main source of vitamin K for most adults. In addition to making vitamins, these bacteria participate in our hormone cycles, transforming some compounds in the bowel and preparing them for absorption back into the blood stream from the colonic mucosa. When these organisms densely colonize the delicate mucosal lining of the bowel, the tissue is healthy because it is protected and because they live in harmony with each other. The mucosa and bacteria actually are beneficial to each other.

A Healthy Barrier is a Necessity

Remember, the original purpose of the gut is for digestion and absorption and keeping things from the outside world from getting absorbed into the blood stream. When the mucosal lining of the bowel is healthy, it becomes a very effective barrier against outside substances getting into the blood stream. There are two main reasons for this. One, the good bacteria make actively anti-microbial substances, so the bacteria themselves help fight invading organisms. Second, when good bacteria are growing on the surface of the colon the colon's cells are healthy, fluffy, and have nice tight junctions between them. These tight junctions create a physical barrier between the blood supplying the mucosal cells and whatever is inside the bowel. Don't forget, these bacteria and the healthy colonic mucosa help the immune system do its job in the gut by fighting invading organisms. So if this topic grosses you out, remember this, if you keep the right bacteria in the colon, you won't have the wrong bacteria growing. If you have the right bacteria growing in the colon, then you'll have a nice, intact barrier that keeps the wrong bacteria away from your blood stream.

When the barrier between the colon and the blood steam is disrupted, then all kinds of junk that is supposed to stay in the colon gets absorbed into the blood stream. The immune system has to fight those organisms in the blood stream and the liver has to detoxify waste products that get absorbed into the blood stream from the colon. The liver's usual mechanism for getting rid of these toxins is to excrete them into the bile and they end up in the intestine again. Toxic compounds can be excreted by the gall bladder and reabsorbed by the colon repeatedly. They go through the cycle from the colon to the blood stream to the liver to the gall bladder to the colon, and then back again. If we do not have good bacteria colonizing the wall of the colon, we will have bad bacteria and fungi (or yeast) living there. These bad organisms cause inflammation, making the barrier more fragile and also opening up the junctions between the cells so that the blood stream has direct exposure to bad organisms and their toxic byproducts.

Prescription Medications

The most common cause I see in my practice for disruption of the barrier between the gut and the blood stream is a history of antibiotic or corticosteroid use. Antibiotics are designed to kill microorganisms, generally bacteria. Most antibiotics are prescribed for infections of other systems, not for infections in the GI tract. My patients have taken antibiotics for respiratory infections or skin infections, etc. These drugs have an effect on the gut ecology. Some of my patients who were on antibiotics years previously still manifest serious abnormalities of gut ecology.

Antibiotics preferentially kill the beneficial species of microbes. This allows bad species that are normally kept in check to multiply and colonize the gut mucosa. When these bad species grow disproportionately large populations, the bowel is stripped of the normal protection afforded by antibiotic properties of the good bacteria. This establishes essentially, a low-grade, long-term, chronic infection in the bowel causing chronic inflammation of the sensitive gut lining. This inflammation of the bowel lining, also known as intestinal permeability, is one cause of many health problems, like: arthritis, asthma, dermatitis, fatigue, food sensitivities, inflammatory bowel disease, etc.

Additionally, these bad bacteria colonizing the gut lining produce toxins that get absorbed into the blood stream. Once in the blood stream our immune system and liver must clean up these toxins. Depending on the species of organism, this process may cause liver damage, kidney damage, nervous system damage, or infections in the blood stream.

The other drug history I see in patients with intestinal permeability is corticosteroids. The most common prescription is Prednisone. These types of steroids change the mucosal cells lining the gut. They cause a thinning of the cells and suppress normal immune function both in the bowel and in the blood stream. These factors set up the gut and the body for infection and latent inflammation that flares up after the corticosteroids are gone.

The thinning of the mucosa by corticosteroids, or the disruption of the good bacteria by corticosteroids and antibiotics predisposes to candida overgrowth. Fungi like candida are everywhere and are normally in the gut in small amounts, but use of antibiotics or corticosteroids can cause the candida to overgrow and colonize the gut lining. Under normal conditions, in the absence of these types of drugs and when the gut is healthy, the immune system can easily keep the candida in check with help from beneficial bacteria that generally colonize the gut lining.

Pause for Review

Hopefully I haven't bored you or grossed you out. I hope the explanation will clarify why I ask folks to do the things that follow in this chapter to keep their digestive tract and bowel functioning properly for long-term health.

Let's review the things that the normal ecology in the bowel creates. A normal environment in the bowel makes vitamins, participates in hormone cycles, fights infections, prevents inflammatory reactions in the blood stream, and helps lower the toxic burden on the liver. Long-term health problems associated with intestinal permeability are chronic and debilitating things like candida or systemic yeast infections, inflammatory arthritis, chronic fatigue, asthma, dermatitis, inflammatory bowel disease, intestinal malabsorption, alcoholism, and food sensitivities.

Food Sensitivities

Next I'd like to talk about food sensitivities. Food sensitivities, or delayed allergic reactions to foods, are one of the most common problems that I see in my office. They cause a myriad of symptoms throughout the body. Almost any disease or symptoms that exist in human beings can be caused by delayed food allergies. This last sentence bears repeating; delayed food allergies can be responsible for almost any symptoms of disease that exist in human beings.

Let me explain the connection between delayed food allergies and the gut. Our immune system has four types of allergic reactions. Type I reactions are the immediate sensitivity reactions. If you have a Type I reaction to food, you will get hives, runny nose, or your throat will close up within about 30 minutes of ingesting the food. But there are three other types of reponses the immune system can mount against a substance. The delayed allergic reactions Type II, III, and IV, take much longer to manifest symptoms because the physiology of the reaction takes longer. The delayed allergies (also known as sensitivities) can take up to three days after ingesting a food for symptoms caused by the immune reaction to manifest. If I eat something on Monday and have a delayed allergic reaction to it, I may not experience symptoms until Wednesday or Thursday. By that time I don't have a clue what I ate Monday, so I would have no way of tracing it back to the food that was the actual offender.

These delayed allergy or sensitivity reactions take place in the blood stream. Let's pick on peanuts. If I eat peanuts and have a high antibody level to peanuts circulating in my blood stream, whenever the peanut protein shows up in my blood stream, my antibodies will combine with that protein. This will set in motion a cascade reaction of the immune system that causes cell destruction anywhere in my blood stream that the original reaction between the peanut protein and the antibody takes place. This is the reason why these types of allergies can cause such a myriad of symptoms. If I have arthritis in my big toe or muscle pain in my neck, when the peanut protein reaches my toe or my neck, the antibodies attack and cause an inflammatory reaction. This inflammatory reaction causes pain and cell destruction in our tissues. Hence, I will have arthritic pain in my toe, or muscle pain and aching in my neck secondary to a food that I ingested.

The key question is, how did the peanut protein get into my blood stream? When I eat, if my stomach and small intestines are functioning properly and if the mucosal membranes of my small and large intestine are intact, then peanut protein should get broken down into small chains of amino acids. These short amino acid chains can't trigger an immune reaction or antibody manufacture by my blood stream. With a healthy properly functioning digestive tract the peanut protein shouldn't get into my blood stream at all. When the digestive tract is healthy the peanut protein is thoroughly broken down in the intestines. A healthy gut lining also protects the immune system in the blood stream from exposure to undigested food proteins. This is why the food sensitivity issue goes back to the health of the digestive tract. This is not true for Type I immediate sensitivities. Type I reactions will still happen regardless of the condition of the GI tract.

Environment for Food Sensitivities

In order for delayed sensitivity reactions to develop, there is a decline of digestion of foods and a deterioration of the health of the mucosal lining of the intestines. Normally with aging, over about forty years old, our stomach makes less stomach acid. Remember, stomach acid is responsible for the beginning phase of protein digestion. Our stomach will also make less pepsin which participates in protein digestion. When we have less stomach acid, we will also have less production and excretion of pancreatic enzymes. The proteins we eat are not getting broken down properly, and digestive function predictably declines the older we get.

The second contributing factor to food sensitivities is any breaks in the intestinal lining. This inflammation of the intestinal lining will expose blood directly to undigested proteins. Even young people with adequate digestion and inflamed mucosal lining will absorb longer chain undigested proteins directly into their blood stream. The immune system will find these undigested proteins in the blood and go on a "seek and destroy" mission for the food proteins, because the immune system is expecting to find bacteria. Again, when this reaction happens and the antibodies combine with the food protein the immune system is tagging as bacteria, white blood cells will join in causing local cell destruction as they try to kill the bacteria. Because there aren't any bacteria, just food protein that provoked the immune reaction, our own body cells are destroyed by our white blood cells.

Anything that causes problems with the ecology in the colon also causes inflammation of the digestive tract lining. Candida problems, which are often secondary to antibiotic use, will cause inflammation of the gut lining and predispose folks to intestinal permeability and food sensitivities. Disruption of the colonic microflora by antibiotic use or disruption of the health of the intestinal lining by corticosteriod use each predispose people to food sensitivities and intestinal permeability. Once people have symptomatic food sensitivities we can test for antibodies to these foods with a blood test. If people eliminate foods the immune system is making antibodies for, then symptoms will usually diminish. I have seen patients with terrible, terrible arthritic pain or tendinitis whose pain almost entirely disappears once they stop eating these foods. If intestinal permeability has progressed enough that the immune system is making antibodies to certain foods, then in order to heal the GI tract, improve the health of the mucosal lining, and improve the ecology in the gut, the offending foods must be eliminated to regain normal function. The measures we will discuss shortly help maintain healthy gut function in folks who are already healthy. Folks I see with altered intestinal permeability have a long slow road back to feeling well again.

Common Signs of Food Sensitivities

When new patients come in to see me, I take an extensive history. There are certain things that are red flags for food sensitivities. Anybody with chronic sinus problems, patients with diabetes, patients with chronic pain, especially arthritis and degenerative arthritis, patients with asthma, and patients with any kind of GI problem, whether it is irritable bowel syndrome, colitis, or indigestion, are all very likely to have elevated antibody levels in their blood to some foods that they are eating on a regular basis.

Common Offending Foods

One of the questions patients frequently ask me is; what are the foods they are most likely to be allergic to? Everyone is concerned they will be allergic to chocolate. Chocolate causes other problems, but I haven't seen any patients with elevated antibodies to chocolate. The most common offending foods I see in my practice are wheat, eggs, and dairy protein. These are the three "biggies".

Wheat

Wheat is a tough one for most people. Wheat products include pasta, breads, cakes, cookies, and anything made with flour. Wheat is hard for people to eliminate because it is a staple of most folks' diet.

Wheat has been hybridized for hundreds of years. The proteins in wheat have a unique potential to irritate the lining of the intestine in many people. I have patients come in with chronic fatigue that is unexplainable. At the intake visit when we set them up for the blood tests etc., I often talk to them about wheat being a problem. When they come back for the results of their blood tests two weeks later they say, "Well, I stopped eating wheat, and you know, I feel much better." That is before they even found out what other foods they have antibodies to.

Antibiotics and Candida

Next, let's talk about candida infection. Antibiotics specifically predispose the gut to overgrowth of candida. When the yeast or candida organisms are growing in the intestines, they are also absorbed into the lymphatic system and the blood stream. They travel from the intestines to the liver and can colonize in the liver, the kidneys, and the spleen. This causes a whole host of symptoms. People with candida will often have fatigue, dizziness, chronic pain, or migratory joint pains. Of course, for women, vaginal yeast infections or chronic bladder infections are common symptoms of yeast infection in the large intestines. This propensity of the yeast organisms to set up housekeeping in other organs like the liver is the reason why chronic candidiasis is so difficult to treat, and why people with candida will have such a variety of symptoms.

Keeping the GI System Healthy

The next topic I would like to talk about is how we get down to the brass tacks of keeping the GI system healthy. The first item is diet. I'm going to repeat what I said on Tape One. The vast volume of what we put into our mouth is the food we eat. If we eat a diet filled with junk food, there is no way we can take enough nutritional supplements to compensate for the volume of junk food we put into our mouths. The best thing we can do for our health is to eat healthy foods. For the GI tract, some of the mechanics of eating are important for good digestion and absorption of food.

Take Time to Chew Thoroughly

The first step in eating is chewing. Food needs thorough chewing so it gets well mixed with enzymes and saliva. This is important for initiating proper digestion of starch. Naturopathic doctors talk about chewing our juices and drinking our foods. What they mean is you want to keep juice in your mouth long enough to expose it well to enzymes and saliva, and chew each mouthful of food long enough that it is liquid once you swallow it.

Regarding the chemistry of eating; if we drink fluids with our meal, we are diluting the stomach acid which makes it less effective. Remember, stomach acid starts the vital protein digestion. For many folks, fluids are better taken toward the end of the meal or after eating. This helps prevent indigestion and bloating.

Relax During Meals

Another thing that we forget in our fast-paced society is that our digestive system is designed to work better if we are relaxed during our meals. We should take time to sit down while we eat. This improves digestion and absorption of food by letting the gut know it can have the time and space to do its job. Our digestive tract works better when our bodies are relaxed. If we are under stress, or in a fight or flight mode, blood gets diverted from the digestive tract. When blood is diverted from the digestive tract it stops what it is doing whether food is present or not. Digestion can be badly impaired by the presence of stress.

Meal Size and Timing

This doesn't mean that we should eat and go to sleep. Eating a large meal before we go to sleep at night is hard on the liver. The liver has to process all the nutrients absorbed into the blood stream from the digestive tract, and, the liver needs rest just like the rest of our body.

Eating a large meal late in the day will predispose the calories to be stored as fat rather than used for energy or production of glycogen, the energy molecule used by muscles. Naturopaths say we should eat breakfast like a queen, lunch like a princess, and dinner like a pauper. Large meals should be taken early in the day and later in the day we should be eating smaller amounts of food. The liver needs to rest at night and our body uses calories more efficiently if they arrive early in the day. Regarding meal size, really large portions of food cannot get adequately digested because they don't get mixed well enough with saliva, stomach acid, pepsin, or the pancreatic enzymes. Our body is not designed to eat very large meals. The normal maximum volume of the stomach, varies from individual to individual. Especially for those habituated to eating large meals the stomach can stretch out. The stomach's normal maximum is about a quart or four cups. We should keep our total meal size, including liquids that we ingest, below the four-cup mark.

Fiber in our Diet

My last topic regarding eating to improve GI function is inclusion of fiber and water. Both fiber and water are extremely important to the function of the large intestine. Once food gets to the large intestine, part of colon function is to absorb water back out of the digested food into the blood stream. If there is not enough water or fiber in our diet to begin with, the digestive matter becomes very solid causing constipation. Fiber in the large intestine has the purpose of holding onto water or bulking up the stool. If you eat fiber, but you don't drink water, the colon and the blood stream will be competing for the water that is available.

The quality of the water and the fiber we ingest is also important. I will talk about problems with water quality later. Not all fibers are created equal. Fiber is essential for normal function in the large bowel, but give up your over-the-counter fiber-in-a-can type products. Please eat your fiber in foods. If you are eating a good diet, you get lots of fiber in your food. Foods that have fiber are fruits, vegetables, seeds, whole grains, and beans.

Remember, fruits and vegetables are also rich in phytonutrients. These are medicinal substances in plants that help our body do its job better. Phytonutrients help the liver work better, they help the immune system work better, they help normalize hormone levels, etc. Vegetables, seeds, cooking herbs, many fruits, and soy products are rich in these wonderful substances.

Whole grains and beans are an excellent source of fiber with the exception of wheat. Remember the proteins in wheat are very irritating to the lining of the small and large intestines in most folks.

Fiber can be soluble or insoluble. The only way to get a large array of both soluble and insoluble fiber is by eating good quality food. Remember, the USDA says we should all be eating five servings of fruits and vegetables daily. I try to get my patients to eat a minimum of two cups of vegetables per day, preferably four. Remember my pet peeve, I beg people not to drown their vegetables in fat. It is best to eat vegetables either lightly steamed, as vegetable juice, salads without dressing, or roasted. Fruits are best eaten fresh or as fresh juice. I try to get people not to eat lots of sugar on their fruit or with their fruit, such as pies, canned fruits in syrup, etc. Sugar in food raises people's blood sugar. Sugar in the GI tract will disrupt the normal balance of the organisms we talked about in the large intestine. This will cause a predisposition to the growth of abnormal bacteria in the colon. In people with candida or a tendency toward candida, sugar will certainly accelerate the candida growth.

Whole Grains

Whole grains and whole beans are a very important part of a healthy diet. Rice is one of the best grains to eat. Rice is hypoallergenic for most people. The ways we eat grains are breads, pasta, and cereals. Please try to get whole grain products. For example, go out of your way to find whole grain pasta. It is important to have all the constituents of the grain present so all the naturally occurring vitamins and minerals are present along with the proteins in the grain. Refining wheat or other grains strips them of protein and essential fatty acids, as well as vitamins and minerals. Remember, we also talked on Tape One about refined grains and their tendency to elevate cholesterol. Refined grains are devoid of fiber and can aggravate or cause constipation. One exception to the preference for whole grains is white rice. For folks who need a hypoallergenic diet (as rice bran is the most allergenic part of rice), white rice is preferable for these sensitive people.

Protein Foods

Large amounts of high protein foods (i.e. meat, poultry, diary products, and fish) cause constipation because these foods are entirely devoid of fiber. Large amounts of protein foods, especially red meat, are hard on the GI tract. These large servings of meat are difficult to digest and also unduly tax the liver and kidneys.

One exception is fish. The fins and scales fish are high in essential fatty acids, and essential fatty acids are important for the health of the mucus membrane and the cells in the intestine that have a high turnover rate. Essential fatty acids decrease inflammation in the gut as well as in other parts of the body. The fins and scales fish, like salmon, halibut, cod, sardines, etc., are actually good to consume and healthy for the GI tract.

Soy foods like tofu and tempeh are high in protein as well as many phytonutrients and soluble fiber. Soy is a much kinder, gentler protein food for our bodies than meats and poultry.

Constipation and Bowel Movements

I would like to talk about constipation and bowel movements. Many of my patients consider they are constipated if they only have one bowel movement every three to four days. Actually, constipation is not having a bowel movement every day. Think about the volume of food you eat and the number of meals. Ideally, we should have one bowel movement for every meal we eat.

In constipation, when the digested food stays in the large intestine for a long period of time, toxic things our body has decided to eliminate in our stool sit against the lining of the large intestine and irritate it. This predisposes people to inflammation of the bowel and/or cancer. Also, the toxic substances in the stool get absorbed into the blood stream and they have to be eliminated another time by the liver into the bile and sent into the intestine again to be eliminated in the stool. This puts an overly difficult burden on the liver to dispose of these substances a second time. What I see in my practice is that if adequate fiber foods and water intake does not eliminate constipation, then probably food sensitivities are involved.

What We Drink Matters

I'd like to talk about fluids other than water. Many people drink coffee and soda. If you're drinking caffeinated beverages, you are actually causing a net loss of fluid from your body. This won't help the large intestine. For patients who drink coffee and soda, I request that they decrease the amount of these beverages. As a minimum request, I want folks to drink an equal amount of water as they do soda pop or coffee.

While we're on the subject of bowel function, either constipation or diarrhea means the colonic environment is abnormal. Some patients live with liquid, watery stools for a long period of time. Any time stools are liquid or watery means there is a gross disruption of the colonic microflora. This needs to be taken seriously and treated properly. I have seen people develop fibromyalgia and chronic arthritis secondary to chronic diarrhea.

Nutrients for the Stomach

My first choice among things that help the stomach work better, is a supplement called "HCl," which stands for hydrochloric acid and pepsin. These usually come together in one product. These factors help the stomach begin to digest protein. If you suspect that you have insufficient stomach acid, you may find that these are helpful for improving digestion in the stomach. If stomach acid is deficient, people really need to supplement with B vitamins, especially B12 and folic acid. Deficits in stomach acid impair the absorption and activity of B vitamins, causing a deficiency of B vitamins. B vitamin deficiency further impairs the manufacture of stomach acid.

This sets up a vicious cycle of declining stomach function. When stomach function declines there is a corresponding decline in digestive function all the way down the line. Other nutrients whose absorption suffers as stomach acid declines are iron and calcium. Appropriate doses for supplementation of some nutrients important for the stomach are: zinc should be supplemented at 15 mg per day, magnesium between 200 and 400 mg per day, vitamin C should be supplemented at 1 to 3 gm per day, beta-carotene at 25,000 IU per day, and calcium should be supplemented between 300 and 800 mg per day. Remember all of these recommendations are for people who are basically healthy and do not have any disease process going on.

Nutrients for the Pancreas

Next down the line in the digestive tract are products to aid pancreatic digestion. These are digestive enzymes. If you shop for supplements that aid digestion, you will see a variety of digestive enzyme products. I steer people toward the vegetable-based digestive enzyme products. The reason is that animal based products will have pancreatin in them. Pancreatin can create a dependency on these products. With vegetable-based enzymes, if you discontinue the product, your body will pick up the slack. In some cases, animal-based enzymes can suppress the pancreatic function. I don't like to see people become dependent on any kind of supplementation.

Digestive enzymes should contain lipase for digestion of fat, amylase for digestion of starches, protease for digestion of protein, and cellulase for digestion of fiber. I don't suggest a dose in milligrams because the potency of enzymes is measured in activity units of the product (i.e. how much protein that enzyme can digest.) I have people take one to two tablets or capsules per meal. Various products will vary greatly in their efficacy. If you try a bottle of something and you don't notice any improvement in how you feel with it, purchase a different product the second time around. Another very potent digestive enzyme is bromelain. This is a concentrated pineapple enzyme product that helps digest proteins.

Time-Honored Digestive Aids

There are a variety of other time-honored digestive aids. These include diluted lemon juice or diluted cider vinegar before meals, bitter herbs like gentian or dandelion, and carminative herbs like ginger, cumin, anise, and cilantro. The bitter herbs can be used to stimulate bile and stomach acid production. Many carminative herbs are common aromatic spices used in cooking. Carminative herbs aid digestion in the small intestine.

There are a variety of herbs that help sooth inflammation in the digestive tract. These are herbs like licorice root, slippery elm, and comfrey. These herbs are generally used as teas. The dosage when making a tea is one tablespoon of herb to one cup of water. When making herb teas, leaves and flowers should be steeped just like you would with a tea bag. When making medicinal tea from roots, they should be boiled for 5 to 10 minutes in order to extract the active compounds from the root into the tea water.

Nutrients for the Intestinal Lining - L-Glutamine

The next group of supplements we'll talk about is the largest group for the GI tract. These are supplements that help the intestinal lining and the small and large intestine. I have two personal favorites based on my experience with patients. One is L-glutamine. L-glutamine is an amino acid that helps regenerate healthy intestinal mucosa cells. The cells lining the intestine have a high turnover rate and use more L-glutamine than any other cells in the body. Providing L-glutamine to these cells helps the new cells be healthier. L-glutamine is used more rapidly any time we are under physical stress. Providing L-glutamine when there is intestinal inflammation can be very good. Incidentally, L-glutamine is used intravenously with patients who are hospitalized with severe ulcerative colitis, because L-Glutamine helps regenerate the mucosal lining of the small and large intestines. I usually start folks with 2 gm of L-glutamine per day, but I've seen benefit with doses as low as 500 mg per day.

Flaxseed

The second of my favorite supplements for the intestinal lining is flaxseed. You have probably heard about flaxseed oil. Folks often don't know flaxseed isn't much use unless it is ground. The seeds are small enough and hard enough that we can't break them with our teeth. The optimal use of flaxseed is as freshly ground seed. The easiest way to grind the seeds is with an electric coffee or spice grinder. Once ground, eat the flax seed within a few minutes (or freeze it in an airtight container) because the essential fatty acids deteriorate rapidly with exposure to air.

Freshly ground flaxseed supplies essential fatty acids which help decrease inflammation and allergic reactions. Essential fatty acids help modulate problems with food sensitivities and delayed allergic reactions. The essential fatty acids in flaxseed also help provide a healing, soothing nutrient for the lining of the intestine.

Flaxseed provides both soluble and insoluble fiber. In addition, the soluble fiber in flax preferentially nourishes the bifidobacter populations in the colon. Different species of beneficial bacteria provide different benefits in the colon. Remember, the colon's function in vitamin manufacture, helping with hormone cycles, helping provide substances the liver needs, and helping provide natural antibiotic activity? Bifidobacter provides multiple functions to aid colon health, and flax fiber's ability to specifically nourish bifidobacter populations may be why it is so useful clinically.

If folks tend toward either constipation or diarrhea, flaxseed fiber can often maintain normal function of the bowel by normalizing either constipation or diarrhea. The dose of flaxseed is one to three tablespoons per day of the freshly ground powder. You can certainly use more if you choose.

Good Bugs

The next class of supplements we'll discuss that benefits intestinal function are called probiotics. These are supplements that contain living beneficial microflora for the intestine. There are several useful species. Most of us have heard of acidophilus. Acidophilus or Lactobacillus acidophilus is present in yogurt that has live cultures. Acidophilus was one of the first beneficial species of bacteria to be used supplementally. Another beneficial supplemental species is bifidobacter that I just mentioned above. There are several other beneficial species. When shopping for a probiotic product, because there are many beneficial species, a product with multiple species usually works better than a single species product. However, the most important factor in any probiotic product, regardless of bacterial species, is that the product delivers live bacteria when you ingest it. Check for this on the label when you buy it. Also, most probiotic products require refrigeration to keep the organisms viable.

Dosage of probiotic supplements is usually half a teaspoon per day of powder or one to two capsules per day. This should provide an adequate maintenance dose.

Patients often tell me they take many doses of acidophilus to keep their health problem at bay, i.e. urinary tract infections, sinus infections, or gastrointestinal problems. This is a sign they have health troubles with their intestinal lining. With each probiotic dose, the numbers of the organism increase temporarily. The good bacterial populations drop back down because the environment in the large intestine is inhospitable for them to take hold and grow. I recommend low doses to my patients because they use probiotic supplements with things like L-glutamine, ground flaxseed, and dietary changes that help heal the large intestine and improve the environment. When they are take probiotic supplements, the small amounts of bacteria are able to attach to the gut lining and multiply to form colonies.

Essential Fatty Acids

Another class of supplements that help maintain normal intestinal function are essential fatty acids. These are extremely useful for any inflammation, including intestinal. Essential fatty acids also calm down the immune system. My favorite sources of supplemental essential fatty acids are black currant oil and a combination of flax oil with borage oil. Either of these products supply a balance of essential fatty acids. Another source of essential fatty acids is evening primrose oil. Fish oil is a supplemental source of essential fatty acids from fatty tissues of fish. I have people start with three capsules per day. One of the best ways to figure out which of the essential fatty acid combinations is best for an individual is to try a bottle of one type, see how you feel with that, and then switch to another type. You might start with flax-borage, then switch to black currant oil and see if you notice a difference.

Pycnogenol or Proanthocyanidin Compounds

The next supplements for the intestinal lining are pycnogenol or proanthocyanidin compounds. These are extracted from plants like gingko, grape seeds, bilberry, or maritime pine. Quercitin and bioflavonoids are similar compounds.

These pycnogenol compounds are potent antioxidants; they are anti-inflammatory, and help with circulation and the health of the capillary walls (the very tiny blood vessels). Any time I am suspecting chronic inflammation or irritation of the intestinal lining, I will recommend these supplements as well. Dosage of these is two to four capsules per day.

FOS

FOS, or fructo-oligosaccharides is a fiber supplement that specifically nourishes the beneficial species of bacteria in the colon. Supplementation with FOS will increase the number of acidophilus and bifidobacter in the large intestine. I prefer to use FOS in conjunction with probiotics and L-glutamine. However, FOS should not be used by folks with candida or klebsiella infections in the gut.

Suggestions for the Healthy

If you're healthy, but having discomfort or symptoms in your abdomen not caused by disease, you could try experimenting with some of the supplements mentioned in this chapter. Many of my patients have bloating ten minutes to three hours after meals, or mysterious indigestion, gas, or belly cramping, etc. These symptoms often go unnoticed until they're asked about. They are indications that the digestive tract is not functioning at its best.

Dosages I've recommended shouldn't be harmful. Exceptions are if you have diagnosed disease like peptic ulcer disease, gastritis, ulcerative colitis, etc., then do not use these supplements. Please seek out a health care practitioner to prescribe supplements that are right for you and your specific condition. For folks with no diagnosable gastrointestinal disease, experimenting with some of these supplements is fine. I recommend that patients try things for four weeks, you should notice a benefit within that time if the supplement is helpful. As I said on the first tape, if you start a supplement and have new symptoms, the supplement is probably causing them. Discontinue the supplement, you are probably sensitive to it. I have seen products cause almost any symptom imaginable in a few patients.

Multi-Vitamin Multi-Mineral

Not to be neglected when we talk about supplementation for GI tract function, is a good quality multi-vitamin multi-mineral. I recommend this to patients as a baseline to provide antioxidants (vitamin A, beta-carotene, vitamin C, and vitamin E), a substantial dose of all the B Vitamins, reasonable potency of minerals, both macro minerals and trace minerals. Check for selenium and chromium. They are important. There should be at least 15 mg of zinc and at least 250 mg of magnesium. Remember, deficiencies of stomach acid will interfere with absorption of nutrients. As we get to be over 45 to 50 years old, additional supplementation becomes essential to prevent deficiency conditions because of the normal declines that all of us suffer in digestion and absorption of our food.

With that it looks like we have reached the end of this second tape in the Free to Be Well© series. On the third tape I will talk about liver function and detoxification.

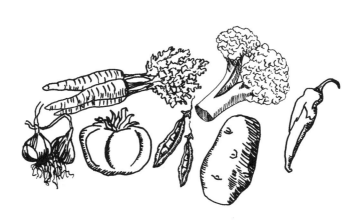

Chapter 3
Leaping Livers

Hello and welcome to Tape Three of the Free to Be Well© series. On this tape, I will be talking about the liver and its vital role in health.

The Role of the Liver

Regarding the liver, I cannot emphasize this topic enough. Many of the conditions I see in my practice (people with diabetes, people with serious neurological conditions, people with immune system problems) their original problems or one of the primary precipitating factors in their disease state goes back to problems with liver function. I hope that I am able to make this topic clear and understandable on this tape.

First of all, what does the liver do? Why do we have a liver? The liver is the largest metabolically active organ in our bodies. It monitors and controls most of our metabolism. The liver is constantly monitoring our blood sugar level so it doesn't get too high or too low. It is constantly monitoring protein in the blood, both albumin and the immune proteins and globulin. The liver is in part responsible for globulin manufacture which are large proteins that are important to immune system function. Much of the immune system is located in the liver. Remember, I said about 50% or more of the immune system is located in the digestive tract in the intestines. Another 25% of the immune system is located in the liver. I will explain why in a little bit.

Another very important function of the liver is monitoring the levels of cholesterol. The liver manufactures cholesterol. Both the good cholesterol (HDL cholesterol) and also the bad cholesterol (LDL cholesterol) are made in the liver. Cholesterol is made by the liver because we need it. It is a very important molecule in our bodies. The liver is also responsible for the levels of triglycerides which are the long-chain fats in our blood stream. The liver is responsible for keeping triglycerides adequate and making sure they do not get too high.

The liver also participates in hormone cycles. Cholesterol is the building block for most of the hormones that occur in our bodies. The liver has to provide cholesterol to our thyroid gland, adrenal glands, etc., so they can make their hormones. The liver also participates in the cycle of those hormones once the molecules get old or the levels get too high. The liver has to figure out how to get rid of those hormones. I see the liver's contribution to hormonal problems in my patients, as the liver is really important in regulating levels of estrogen, progesterone, and testosterone. In my female patients experiencing menopause, many times menopausal symptoms go back to the liver's inability to participate normally in hormone cycles.

How the Liver Works

So, how does the liver do all this? Remember from the second tape that the inside of the digestive tract technically is the outside of the body. In other words, we can eat all manner of things that should not end up in our blood stream, and if we are functioning normally and healthily, they do not end up in our blood stream. How does that happen? First of all, remember, the mucous membrane lining of the GI tract from the mouth to the other end has to be intact to keep what is in the gut isolated from the blood stream, except what the body chooses to absorb. The second thing that happens is that the part of the blood stream that supplies the small and large intestines is kept isolated from the rest of the body until it goes through the liver. The liver has to examine in detail all of the substances that come from the intestines and figure out what to do with them. The liver deals with the foods we eat, in other words the sugars and fats and the proteins and the starches. It transforms them and puts them out into the blood stream in forms that the body can use. It is also examines the blood that comes from the small and large intestines for toxic substances or infectious substances, and the liver has to deal with those. This is why there is so much of the immune system located in the liver and why the liver is responsible for detoxification. The liver's detoxification function is going to be a large part of the subject matter on this tape. Try to remember that *everything* we eat or drink has to be screened and transformed and/or eliminated by the liver.

In addition to examining all of the things that come from the small and large intestines, the liver is also constantly monitoring the blood that comes from the rest of our body. As a normal part of our bodies' functions, toxic substances are created. These toxic substances could be normal metabolic waste products, they could be products from inflammation, or they could be products of the immune system doing its job in the body. Those things end up in the blood stream and have to get cleaned out. They get cleaned out primarily by the liver or the kidneys. When the liver cells detect toxic substances and decide to deal with them, these things go through what is called 'detoxification'. I will talk about that later.

Once the liver transforms these things and makes them into forms it can get rid of, they get collected through tubules in the liver and get sent to the gall bladder in the form of bile. Remember the gall bladder and bile help to digest fat. Bile is also a way for the liver to get rid of toxic things. The bile is a route for the liver to dump transformed toxins into the intestinal tract. When we eat meals and the gall bladder does its contraction thing and squeezes bile out into the small intestines to help with digesting the fatty portion of the meal, we are also dumping toxic substances. This is the reason it is so important not to be constipated; if we are constipated, those toxic substances will get reabsorbed into the circulation in the large intestines and end up in the blood stream. Then the liver ends up having to detoxify them and get rid of them a second time. I hope this provides a window on the physical route of what happens to many of the toxic compounds in our bodies.

Liver Detoxification Pathways

I would like to talk next about the liver's detoxification function and how that happens. This will get into some chemistry, but I will try not to bore you. The liver's detoxification function has two pathways. They are named Phase I and Phase II.

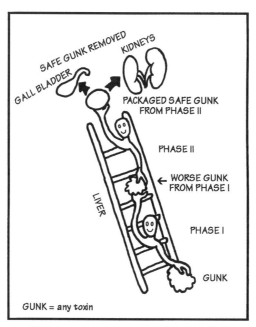

PHASE I and PHASE II DETOX PATHWAYS
IN THEIR HEALTHY STATE

The Phase I pathways are enzyme based and the liver can make more of these enzymes. They are called cytochrome P450 enzymes (if you get into the chemistry.) These cytochrome P450 enzymes can do what is called "up regulate." In other words, the liver can make more of these enzymes so it can speed up the Phase I detoxification pathways. This happens when the liver is regularly presented with a compound that gets detoxified completely or partly by these enzymes.

In the Phase II pathways, the liver cannot up regulate. In other words, whatever shows up for Phase II to deal with, the liver deals with it at the same rate of speed. So if more things show up that need to go through Phase II, the liver does not make Phase II go faster. Toxic things that need to go through Phase II just hang around. They hang around either in liver cells or in the blood stream. As you might guess, some compounds go through Phase I and some compounds go through Phase II, and other compounds need to go through both phases: Phase I and then Phase II.

A few compounds (like caffeine) go through only the Phase I liver detox pathway. Since most people can speed up Phase I, their livers can handle caffeine fairly well.

Problems start when things only go through Phase II or they need to go through Phase I and then Phase II. The Phase II pathways cannot easily speed up. The Phase I detox pathways can readily speed up. In some folks, the liver deals with things in Phase I, but Phase II cannot

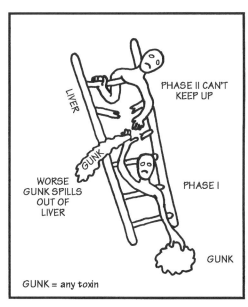

FAILURE OF PHASE II
DETOX PATHWAYS

keep up the pace. Compounds that have been through Phase I but are waiting for Phase II are many times more toxic after they've gone through Phase I than if the liver had left them alone. Those compounds are called toxic intermediates. Because Phase II can't easily speed up, once those toxic intermediates have gone through Phase I and Phase II is not ready for them yet, they build up in the liver cells and then get spilled out into the blood stream. So compounds that started out toxic actually become more dangerous and end up in the blood stream circulating throughout the body. By this mechanism, which is not unusual, problems with the liver's detoxification process become problems adversely influencing our health generally.

When the toxic intermediates that have gone through Phase I but have not been through Phase II yet build up in the blood stream, they tend to get stored in the tissues, especially fatty tissues, so they won't be constantly circulating and damaging cells in the whole body. Fatty tissues they get stored in are endocrine glands such as: breast tissue, thyroid gland, adrenal glands, etc. They also get stored in the nervous system. The brain and spinal cord are storage sites for these toxic intermediates because the brain and spinal cord are mostly fat. You can probably let your imagination run wild about what these compounds can potentially do in these tissues. I will talk about that a little later.

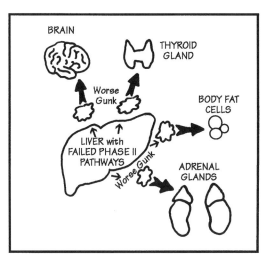

SOME ORGANS WHICH STORE TOXINS
IF LIVER DETOX FAILS

Causes of Decreased Functional Capacity of the Liver

I would like to talk about the causes of the liver losing its functional capacity. From a functional standpoint, the liver's ability is definitely affected throughout our lifetime. The older we get and the more things the liver is exposed to, the more difficult it is for the liver to do its job. The liver is adversely affected in its functional capacity by alcohol use, especially regular alcohol use. It is also affected by hepatitis. If you have ever had hepatitis, that will affect your liver's ability to deal with things. If you have ever been in a starvation state from lack of food (voluntarily or involuntarily) that will affect the liver and in many cases will affect the liver permanently. That is one of my pet peeves with the extremely low calorie diets — starvation diets — are extremely bad for the liver.

Starvation

I mentioned starvation and am serious when I say that low-calorie diets put the body into a starvation state. This is very dangerous for the liver. There are many other health problems with low-calorie diets, and I will get into that on another tape.

Toxins in the Gut

Things that can overload the liver's detox capacity include toxins from the gut. Remember from the second tape when I was talking about all the problems with the ecology in the large intestine? When you have the wrong mix of bacteria colonizing the large intestine, when you have any kind of inflammation on the lining of the large intestine, or if you have chronic yeast infection in the large intestine, all of those things will increase the toxic burden being absorbed by the blood stream from the intestines. Remember, that blood goes from the intestines straight to the liver so the liver has to deal with all these things.

Toxins we Eat or Drink

Any toxins in the things we eat or drink get absorbed into the blood stream. These could be bacteria, viruses, alcohol, preservatives in foods, the bad fats that we eat, especially if the fats are rancid or hydrogenated (these are very toxic), and residues of farming chemicals. Refined sugars are difficult for the liver because refined sugars require B vitamins and magnesium in order to be metabolized in the liver. The liver needs B vitamins and magnesium to do other things, and refined sugar will deplete those biochemical pathways of their B vitamins and magnesium - essentially stealing resources from other jobs.

The liver has to deal with residues of pesticides and herbicides that are used on crops. Other toxins in our foods are the antibiotics that are fed to poultry and beef, and hormones that are given to poultry and beef. The liver needs to be able to detoxify those compounds and they place an undue burden on liver function. Additionally, in our foods we get residues from the packaging materials. These are residues from plastic that the foods sit up against and residues from aluminum. These compounds also need to be dealt with by the liver. In our water supply we have microbes and chemicals. The organisms go straight to the liver and the chemicals in drinking water go straight to the liver. The liver again has to figure out what to do with these things.

Drugs

Another source of liver damage is drugs. I do not care whether we are talking about prescription drugs, over-the-counter drugs, or recreational drugs; they are all potentially toxic to the liver. There are a few drugs that are primarily dealt with by the kidneys, and those can be problematic for the kidneys and not for the liver. Most medications that we use, no matter whether they are recreational, over-the-counter, or prescription, are toxic to the liver to some extent.

Certainly, some compounds are much more toxic than others. As I said, caffeine primarily goes through the Phase I liver detox pathway and caffeine tends to be much less toxic for most people than other kinds of drugs we could be using. If someone has trouble with the Phase I pathways (each of us is biochemically individual and everyone is different) then caffeine will likely make you very uncomfortable.

When it comes to drugs, some of the ones that bother me the most when patients come in and say they are taking drugs, are those used for indigestion such as Tagamet and Pepcid AC. They are in the class of H2 blockers. The other worrisome over-the-counter drug is acetaminophen, also known as Tylenol. This drug depletes nutrients necessary for more than one of the Phase II liver detox pathways. Acetaminophen used in combination with either alcohol or garden chemicals can cause very serious permanent liver damage and/or need for a liver transplant. Another class of drugs that are very hard on the liver are steroid hormones, Prednisone, etc. If you are familiar with the corticosteroids such as Prednisone, I probably don't need to mention all the other problems Prednisone causes in the rest of the body. But Prednisone puts a greatly increased burden on the liver to eliminate it from the blood stream.

Chemicals

Another group of toxins that are dangerous for the liver are synthetic chemicals. Just about anything that is a product of chemical manufacturing should be suspect. We are usually exposed to these chemicals through breathing them; and if you can smell a compound in the air, you are getting enough of it absorbed into your blood stream when you breathe that it will affect your liver. You can also be exposed to these compounds through your skin. Many of these things will get absorbed through the skin. For example, farm workers need to be very careful when they are mixing and using herbicides, pesticides, and organophosphate compounds because they can absorb enough through the skin to actually cause permanent neurological damage or even death.

The typical folks I see with very high chemical exposure in my practice are people who have worked in the construction industry, in furniture refinishing, painters, and people who work in certain types of manufacturing where they are using lots of chemicals.

Signs of Decreased Liver Function

Once we have had ongoing exposure to any of the things I mentioned above, what can we expect as far as liver function? Every person is an individual. We all have a unique appearance, we all have unique personalities, and we also have unique biochemistry. Therefore, what may be true for one person in terms of their threshold of illness based on toxic exposure, is not going to be true for the next person. Remember, these toxic intermediate compounds tend to build up in the body and get stored in tissues, and that causes symptoms that people notice.

Fibromyalgia and Chronic Fatigue Syndrome

Fibromyalgia and Chronic Fatigue Syndrome are often related to poor liver detox function. A build up of toxic intermediates in tissues can affect our mitochondria. Mitochondria are little energy factories that we have in every single one of our cells, so when these compounds are circulating in the blood stream, it affects the ability of our cells to make energy. Many people feel this in their muscles, this is fibromyalgia. Many people feel this as fatigue, which is chronic fatigue syndrome. The cases I see in my practice of either fibromyalgia or chronic fatigue syndrome have either a primary problem with the liver detox pathways or a secondary problem with the liver detox pathways.

Balance, Headaches, and Mood

Balance problems often go back to problems with the liver, because the toxic intermediates like to be stored in fatty tissue like the brain and spinal cord. When they are stored in the spinal cord or in certain brain centers, people will develop trouble with their balance.

Many folks get headaches with exposure to toxic chemicals. For example, if someone walks through the room wearing perfume and you have to breathe that for a few minutes and end up getting a headache,

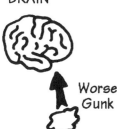

BRAIN

Worse Gunk

that says that your liver detox pathways are not up to snuff. The perfume gets into your bloodstream in the air you breathe and your liver has to get it out of your blood. If your liver can't keep up, you get a headache. If you get a headache when you go into a place that has new carpeting, that is also a sign that your liver detox pathways are not working well enough.

Problems with mood, depression or manic depression often are caused by a build up, again, of the toxic intermediates in the brain. There are many other things that can cause problems with mood or depression, so this is not always the mechanism here, but it can be. When seizure disorders onset late in adulthood, the first thing I ask about is their history of toxic chemical exposure. Many times these people do have a history of exposure to toxic chemicals. If people have seizure disorders that start in childhood, this does not usually point to a problem with the liver detox pathways.

Neurological Diseases, PMS, and Cancer

Many types of neurological diseases, especially the ones that onset later in life such as multiple sclerosis and Parkinson's disease, often have a history of toxic chemical exposure. There have been several cases reported in literature of people in their thirties developing Parkinson's disease after a combination of recreational drug use and chemical exposure on the job.

Many kinds of endocrine problems have at their root, or as a significant contributing factor, problems with the liver's ability to detoxify things. In my practice I see PMS, difficult periods where women have terrible cramping and heavy bleeding, or problems with menopause that go back to some problem with liver function.

The last thing I would like to mention here is cancer. Many scientists and clinicians are becoming more and more aware of the fact that a problem with the liver's Phase II detox pathways can contribute to cancer. I will talk to this more when we discuss cancer on Tape Six.

There are numerous other symptoms or diseases that people develop because of decreased functional ability of the liver's detox pathways, but these are the most common conditions related to liver dysfunction.

Consequences Seen in my Practice

I would like to give some examples I see clinically when the liver is involved. One scenario is very rapid weight loss, whether one has stopped eating because of emotional problems or is engaging in a fitness regimen with dieting, exercise, and rapid weight loss. Remember the body likes to store these toxic chemicals in fatty tissues. This includes the fat cells of the body. When fatty tissues are rapidly lost, then these chemicals are liberated in a large volume all at once into the blood stream. This causes a sudden re-exposure of the body and the liver to large amounts of toxins. Generally people who have a history of toxic exposure and then lose a lot of weight will, sometime within six months to two years of that weight loss, develop some serious disease like seizures, neurological problems, or chronic fatigue syndrome.

An example that many people have heard is the Vietnam War veterans who were exposed to dioxin and decided to, some years later, get on a weight loss program and exercise and after that time had children with birth defects. This was because of the effects of the dioxin on the sperm. In many cases these veterans also developed chronic fatigue syndrome.

Another scenario that I see in practice is people who have extreme weight gain subsequent to things that would cause liver problems. This could be extreme weight gain after a large exposure to toxic chemicals or extreme weight gain after having had hepatitis or another liver disease. Another example I see is people with diabetes who have abnormal liver detoxification function. For each of these folks, often improving the functional ability of the liver to do its detoxification pathways normally and improving the ecology of the gut with nutritional therapies will greatly improve their blood sugar control. Folks with fibromyalgia, chronic fatigue, or migraine headaches who do liver treatment and treatment for the ecology of the colon can see their symptoms diminish greatly or even vanish.

I would like to briefly discuss neurological disorders. I do see patients with serious neurological disorders who have a history of toxic exposure to chemicals and/or heavy metals. Principle among the heavy metals is mercury. If you are not aware of it, mercury is a very toxic substance to the nervous system. A lot of my patients ask, "Where the heck did I get mercury?", and I say, "Do you have any of those silver fillings in your teeth?" If silver fillings are more than 15-18 years old, they leach significant amounts of mercury every time you chew, brush your teeth, or drink hot liquids. Mercury and other toxic metals also remain in our bodies for decades and many of my patients in their forties and older who have elevated mercury levels played with mercury as kids.

Case Study

I would like to give a case study from my practice. This patient was approximately 39-years-old when she first came to me with serious neurological problems. She had a lot of problems with her balance and was unable to run. She had great difficulty climbing stairs and had difficulty walking long distances. With stair climbing and walking she had extreme fatigue in her lower extremities. She had been worked up by the medical doctors, and their initial diagnosis was multiple

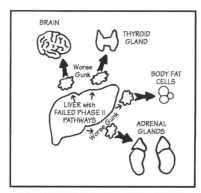

SOME ORGANS WHICH STORE TOXINS
IF LIVER DETOX FAILS

sclerosis. I asked a lot of questions and the M.D.'s amended their diagnosis to a demyelinating disorder of the spinal cord. The medical prognosis was that this woman would be in a wheelchair in less than six months and that she would lose the ability to use her lower extremities. I did my standard evaluation with her which included a hair mineral analysis and liver detox profile and found that several of the liver detox pathways were abnormal and she had elevated levels of mercury in her hair. When I explained to her that mercury is a neurotoxin, she chose to have all of the silver amalgam fillings in her mouth replaced with gold. I also started her on aggressive nutritional therapies to help improve her liver detox function, to help improve the environment of the large intestine, and to help her liver rid her body of the toxic chemicals she had been exposed to.

It was approximately three years ago that she had the mercury removed from her teeth and we started on an aggressive liver detox nutritional supplementation regimen. The progression of her spinal cord disease stopped. She never lost the use of her legs, and about six months ago this patient had a dramatic improvement in her ability to balance. She also began to be able to run short distances and walk long distances again. At this time this particular patient works out on a treadmill, a combination of walking and running, twenty minutes daily.

This is an example of someone who the medical industry basically wrote off and told her to forget about it, you're going to lose your legs in six months. By watching her diet really carefully and taking nutritional supplements, this patient has not only halted the progression of her spinal cord disease, but she has started to reverse the deterioration and has regained a significant portion of her previous normal function.

Appeal to Folks with Neurological Diagnoses

I relate this story as an appeal to people who may be listening to this tape series who have been diagnosed with a disease like multiple sclerosis, Parkinson's, or some other serious spinal cord or neurological disease. I beg of you, please do not consider that the diagnosis you have been given will lead inevitably to deterioration. On the other hand, you must understand that, once your neurological disease has progressed to the point that the medical doctors have enough evidence to give you a diagnosis, it will be a long, slow recovery. It will take a lot of work on your part to be very careful, always vigilant about what kinds of food you eat, always taking the appropriate nutritional supplementation to help improve your body's metabolism, keeping active as much as you can, and having faith in your body's amazing ability to heal itself!

Decreasing the Liver's Work Load

This brings me to my next subject. Once people have a disease that is serious enough to be diagnosed and is related to problems with the liver detoxification pathways, just normal metabolism becomes problematic for that person's liver. In other words, we are always making toxic things inside our body that the liver has to eliminate. These things are byproducts of the immune system, byproducts of hormone metabolism, byproducts of cellular metabolism; just the normal waste products of our body. Our liver has enough to cope with between what comes in normally in our food and what is made inside our bodies. This is why the healing process for some of these serious diseases such as chronic fatigue syndrome and fibromyalgia and serious neurological diseases is so slow. It is because the body has to keep doing its thing and the liver has to keep being able to get rid of the toxins that are part of its normal daily load. Once we start it on the healing road and improve its detox ability, the liver can start lowering that total toxic burden that has accumulated over years or decades of life in the body tissues.

Imagine the liver is buried under this massive dump of stuff and is trying to clean itself out. This is why I am so strict with patients about further exposure to anything hazardous. On that hazardous list of things, we need to include household cleaning products. Things like bleach are extremely toxic to the liver and to all of our cells. You know what bleach does to any surfaces and clothing that it comes in contact with? Well it does the same thing to our cell membranes. When bleach contacts cell membranes, it destroys them which means it kills the cells it comes in contact with. The chlorine from bleach gets absorbed into our blood stream by breathing it. If you can smell the bleach in the air, you are getting bleach into your blood stream and it is coming in contact with your cells. Please be very cautious of any kind of household cleaners or other kinds of products that have warning labels on them. This is an indication that they are potentially toxic to the liver. There are more and more household cleaning products and other products that we can use that are ecologically safe and also nontoxic to us.

Food Categories to Avoid

Let's talk about how the foods we eat can help keep our livers healthy and thereby keep the rest of our body healthy and feeling well. The number one item; please do not eat bad fats. These are margarine, hydrogenated oil, corn oil, cotton seed oil, and rancid oils and fats. All of these fats are extremely toxic to the liver and should be considered unfit to eat. Remember to check the ingredient labels on foods that you buy to make sure that none of these fats are present. Hydrogenated oils are particularly ubiquitous and tend to be present in many foods that you find in the supermarket.

The second group of foods to avoid are those that are high in pesticides, herbicides, and other agricultural chemical residues. Whenever possible try to eat organically grown produce and grains. If this is not possible, there are some crops that tend to be especially high in toxic chemical residues. For these foods, please do your best to get them organically grown. That list includes apples, apricots, bell peppers, celery, cherries, grapes (remember raisins and wines are made from grapes), peaches, spinach, strawberries, wheat, green beans, and peanuts. Please try to get these foods in their organically grown counterparts.

The third category of foods to avoid is those that include antibiotics and hormone residues. These are toxic and these compounds tax our liver's detox capacity. Foods that contain antibiotics and hormone residues are meats, dairy, and poultry. As much as possible try to purchase organically raised free-range meats and poultry and organic dairy products.

When you go to the store and look for these organically raised grains, fruits, vegetables, meats, and dairy products, you may find they are a bit more expensive than their counterparts in the regular supermarket. The more consumers demand these kinds of foods, the more the prices will come down on the organically raised foods. Organically raised foods are important not just for improving liver detox pathways, but also in preventing allergic reactions to food and preventing cancer.

Other toxic things that we get in our food supply are artificial colors, preservatives, artificial sweeteners, and other chemical additives. These compounds are not good for us, do not occur naturally, and place an undue burden on our livers to eliminate. Please avoid foods that have these kind of chemical additives in them.

Cooking Methods to Avoid

Charbroiling meats creates chemicals that put an increased burden on the liver detox pathways. This is not a good way to cook meats. Another cooking method that creates free radicals and other toxic compounds is deep frying with very hot oil. Whenever oil gets so hot that it is smoking, toxic compounds are created in the oil. Cooking methods like charbroiling meat and smoking frying oil are a source of toxic compounds.

More Food Categories to Avoid

The next category of foods to avoid for liver health are grains and flours that have been refined. The refining process of grains strips the minerals and naturally occurring vitamins, and these things are needed by the liver to do its job. When you eat refined foods, in essence, they will deplete the liver of minerals and vitamins. Refined sugars do the same thing to the liver by depriving it of nutrients that it needs. Fortification of white flour, in other words wheat flour that has been stripped of its bran and germ and then fortified with iron and a couple of B vitamins, is not nearly as nutritious as organically raised whole wheat flour that has not been stripped of nutrients. The refining process of wheat strips away about twenty nutrients from the wheat and fortification adds back less than ten.

Foods to Eat for a Healthy Liver

Now that I have told you what not to eat, let's talk about what you should eat. In short, a brief summary of what to eat includes a lot of fruits, a lot of vegetables, whole grains, soy products, especially tofu and/or tempeh, fresh fish (remember this is your fins and scales type fish such as salmon, sardines, halibut, cod, etc.)

Following that very brief summary, I would like to go into more detail beginning first with vegetables. One of the big buzz words I am sure you have heard is phytonutrients or the term nutraceuticals. These are terms for naturally occurring compounds that help the body with its own normal biochemistry and normal metabolism. "Phyto" means plant, so phytonutrients are nutrients from plants. Beta-carotene and carotenoid compounds are one class of phytonutrients. Pycnogenol type compounds are another class of phytonutrients. There are many beneficial groups of phytonutrients that have been studied and more are being discovered all the time.

Vegetables

Vegetables are one of the groups of foods that are very high in phytonutrients. The first vegetable family we will discuss is the cabbage family. The cabbage family is high in sulfur and also in phytonutrients that aid the liver's Phase II detox pathways. Remember that Phase II is very hard to normalize if it becomes depressed, which it often does, especially in people with various types of illnesses. The cabbage family of vegetables can actually help improve the liver's Phase II pathways which can be extremely beneficial to health. The cabbage family of vegetables includes vegetables like broccoli, kale, cauliflower, cabbage, bok choy, collard greens, and Brussels sprouts. I try to get my patients to eat one cup of this group of vegetables per day.

A second group of vegetables high in sulphur compounds which will help the liver's Phase II detox pathways is the onion family. This would be all of the onion varieties and also the various garlics.

Another group of phytonutrients are found in the red, yellow, orange class of vegetables. They are rich in the carotenoid compounds. You have probably heard of beta-carotene. Beta-carotene is only one of a variety of carotenes which are called carotenoids generally. All of the yellow, orange, red vegetables, like tomatoes, yams, carrots, beets, and many of the various squashes, are rich in the carotenoids and various other phytonutrients that help the liver's Phase I detox pathways. Parsley is also very beneficial for liver function.

Soy

Another class of foods that is extremely rich in phytonutrients and phytosterols (phytosterols means plant hormones) are soy and soy products. Some of the nutrients in soy are unavailable unless the soy has been made into either tofu or tempeh. Tempeh is a fermented soybean product and tofu is the bean curd or the curdled protein portion of soy milk. On Tape One we heard that soy also helps normalize cholesterol levels.

Calcium without Milk

I discourage many of my patients from using dairy because so many people are allergic to it or sensitive to it. One of the questions I am commonly asked is, "Where am I going to get my calcium if I'm not drinking milk?" Here are some alternative foods that are high in calcium. Tofu, if it is curdled with a calcium mineral salt, is high in calcium. Broccoli and kale are also excellent sources of calcium. A note on calcium absorption and retention with a diet high in protein: in order for the kidneys to deal with the protein in your diet, they will send calcium out in your urine. Dairy products *are* high in calcium, but because dairy also is high in protein, many people have a net loss of calcium if they depend on dairy for their calcium intake. One advantage of getting calcium from broccoli and kale is that these groups are very low in protein which means the calcium in broccoli and kale will be retained.

Fruits

The next group of foods that I recommend are fruits. A fruit that helps the liver's function are grapes, especially red and concord varieties (any reddish or purplish grapes are rich in pycnogenol compounds.) These pycnogenols or proanthocyanadin compounds are very potent antioxidants which help the liver do its job much more easily. Remember when we are talking about grapes to look for organically raised grapes rather than grapes that are high in chemical residues that will undo the benefit of eating the grapes. Apples also contain a variety of beneficial phytonutrients and they have soluble fiber which helps the liver maintain normal cholesterol levels. Remember that apples are another one of those fruits that you want to get organically grown. Blueberries help normalize blood sugar.

Many people are sensitive or allergic to citrus, so those folks should not be consuming citrus. If citrus does not bother you, lemons, limes, and oranges are rich in a variety of beneficial compounds. Do not use grapefruit regularly though, as it has naringenin which is a compound that inhibits the liver's Phase I enzyme pathway. Occasional use of grapefruit is fine. Pineapple is another beneficial fruit. Pineapple and papaya are both rich in enzymes that aid with digestion which will make the liver's job easier.

This is by no means a complete list of beneficial fruits. I picked out highlights among fruits I am aware of in the scientific literature. If you have some fruit that is a favorite of yours, like bananas or peaches, feel free to consume it as it is likely benefitting you. Remember science has a long way to go before it discovers even the tip of the iceberg in this area.

Whole Grains

Whole grains are an important part of a good diet that benefits the liver. Grains are rich in minerals that help the liver do its job, and they are also rich in both soluble and insoluble fiber which will help keep the intestine healthy and help the liver regulate cholesterol levels. It is important to eat a variety of grains. Many people develop a sensitivity to grains, especially if their diet is based on one grain, like wheat. If you eat mainly bread and pasta, try branching out. Eat rice or rice pasta a few times a week. Try cooking quinoa for breakfast or dinner. Quinoa is an ancient grain with a mildly nut-like flavor. It is higher in protein than other grains.

Proteins

You will notice that I have not really talked about protein foods, and I am not going to either. Protein is important for the liver in that we must get an adequate amount, but most people in North America eat much more protein than they need. An adequate amount for most people is about 4 oz. of meat, fish, or poultry per meal. If the protein you are relying on is tofu or soy, then 7 oz. per meal should be enough. Dairy products are almost as protein dense as meat products, therefore, 4-5 ounces of dairy products is plenty per meal. Protein needs to be metabolized by the liver when it comes from the gastrointestinal tract, so a diet high in protein will tax the liver's ability to cope with its normal work load. A diet high in protein also taxes the kidneys as they do their job, so folks with any kidney problem should eat a diet low in protein.

Nutrients that Help Liver's Phase I Function

Now that we've covered a basic diet for the liver, let's move on to the nutrients that help the liver do a better job. The first category is nutritional supplements that help the liver's Phase I pathways. These are principally antioxidant type supplements. Typical antioxidants are: beta-carotene, vitamin C, vitamin E, lipoic acid, and herbs like milk thistle and gingko. Dosages for these: I generally recommend between 25,000 and 50,000 IU per day of beta-carotene; about 2,000 mg per day vitamin C, and 400 IU of vitamin E. I recommend a minimum of 100 mg per day of lipoic acid, to be taken with food. Herbs like milk thistle and gingko generally come in capsule products and I suggest that people take 2-4 capsules of those herbs per day. Gingko contains pycnogenol type compounds which are very potent antioxidants. Milk thistle (aka Silybum marianum) is an antioxidant herb specific for the liver.

Nutrients that Help Liver's Phase II Function

The next group of supplements are nutrients that help the liver's Phase II detox pathways do a better job. These are primarily the sulphur-bearing amino acids. Remember the cabbage family and onion family are rich in sulphur. Vegetables from these families help the Phase II pathways primarily. The sulphur-bearing amino acids also help the liver's Phase II pathways. Amino acids are the building blocks of protein, and there are specific amino acids that contain a sulphur group. The liver uses the sulphur group from the sulphur-bearing amino acids to attach to toxic compounds that it is trying to eliminate. These sulphur-bearing amino acids are taurine, methionine, reduced glutathione, cysteine, and N-acetyl cysteine. In order for amino acids to get properly absorbed, they should be taken on an empty stomach. (If they cause stomach upset, take them with a small amount of carbohydrate like bread or a rice cake.) I usually have my patients take 1000 mg per day of taurine or methionine. Reduced glutathione dose is about 500 mg per day. For cysteine and N-acetyl cysteine, I usually recommend 500 to 1000 mg per day.

I would like to note a caution regarding the sulphur-bearing amino acids. Please, if you have any condition like MS, Parkinson's, or any mysterious neurological disease, or high levels of mercury in your body, do not take methionine, cysteine, or N-acetyl cysteine, also known as NAC. These amino acids could actually worsen your condition, so *please don't* use them if you have any of the conditions I just mentioned. For patients in my practice who do have those conditions and need sulphur-bearing amino acids, taurine does not have the kind of side effects that these other amino acids have.

Giving your Liver the Basics

The lists above of nutrients for the Phase I and II pathways are by no means complete lists of nutrients for the liver. The liver must have a base dose for many of its metabolic pathways of a variety of nutrients. Before you consider giving the liver the fancy stuff, I always ask my patients to give the liver the basics it needs to do its job properly. The place to start with the basics for the liver is a good quality multi-vitamin multi-mineral. The liver needs all the macro minerals and trace minerals as well as antioxidants and B vitamins for so many of its processes that a good quality multi-vitamin multi-mineral is the baseline in proper nutritional support. I will talk later on this tape about how to chose a good quality nutritional supplement.

Multi-Vitamin Multi-Mineral

When you do find that supplement, make sure you check the label to see how many tablets or capsules the manufacturer recommends that you take per day. A good quality supplement will state on the label that you need to take from 4-8 tablets or capsules per day in order to get the listed dose on the label of the minerals and vitamins. Some of the minerals to look for are magnesium, calcium, zinc, chromium, selenium, manganese, boron, and iodine. A good quality product will be available in two versions, one with iron and one without iron. If you do not know your iron status, you should pick a product that has less than 10 mg of iron per day.

All the antioxidants are important for basic liver function. Those are vitamin C, vitamin A, beta-carotene, vitamin E, and lipoic acid. If you aren't familiar with lipoic acid, it is a very potent antioxidant and it helps the body recycle beta-carotene, vitamin C, and vitamin E. You will get two to three times the mileage out of your other antioxidants when you are using lipoic acid as a supplement. Remember to take lipoic acid with food, not on an empty stomach, to avoid low blood sugar. All of the B vitamins are really important for liver function, so make sure you are getting the full spectrum of B vitamins in adequate doses.

Essential Fatty Acids

A supplement that is commonly forgotten is the essential fatty acids. These are extremely important for liver function and are virtually absent from the modern diet. Essential fatty acids are vital for proper cholesterol metabolism in the liver. They help keep cholesterol from getting too high. The main source of essential fatty acids in the modern diet is fish (remember your fins and scales type fish such as salmon, halibut, cod, and sardines.) In order to get enough essential fatty acids from only fish, you need to have four servings per week of these types of fish. If you aren't that much of a fish eater, then you will want to get essential fatty acids in the form of a nutritional supplement; such as oils from plants. Look for flax oil, a combination of flax and borage, black currant oil, or evening primrose oil. I have my patients experiment with the various products and see which one they feel the best on. Once you find something that you feel good on, you should take two to four capsules per day. These essential fatty acid supplements are also useful as anti-inflammatories. You can take them in higher doses to prevent inflammation.

Phosphatides

The next group of supplements that are important for basic liver function are the phosphatides. These have very long names, phosphatidyl choline, phosphatidyl inositol, and phosphatidyl ethanolamine. These have been shown to protect the liver. They also help improve the quality of cell membranes throughout the body which is very important in preventing inflammation and improving cellular function. They help prevent gall stones from forming and phosphatides help improve the function of the central nervous system and mental function. The baseline dose for these if you chose to supplement with them is 300 to 500 mg per day. These can be difficult to find. They are present in lecithin which is extracted from soy. Lecithin products should say on the label how much of these phosphatides they contain, so you can figure out your milligrams of phosphatides based on the lecithin label if you can't find the phosphatides themselves.

Benefits of Good Gastrointestinal Health

The last group of supplements that I would like to talk about for the liver are nutrients that aid the liver by improving the state of gastrointestinal health. These are L-Glutamine, which we talked about on a previous tape, and also freshly ground flaxseed. Recall that L-Glutamine helps maintain good health of the intestinal lining cells, thus helping to prevent inflammatory byproducts from the intestines getting into the blood stream and taxing the liver. Freshly ground flaxseed helps maintain a normal mix of bacteria in the large intestine, which also helps prevent inflammatory byproducts from crossing into the blood stream.

The normal bacterial flora in the large intestine produce compounds that help the liver do its job better when these things get absorbed

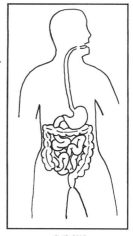

THE GUT

into the blood stream from the large intestine. Normal bacterial flora help prevent reabsorption of compounds that the liver excretes in the bile. The liver gets rid of things in the bile and they are passed out in the stool if the bacterial flora in the colon is normal. Normal bacterial flora in the colon will help prevent colon cancer.

Making Better Choices

The last thing I would like to talk about regarding the liver is some of the things you should not do. Alcohol, especially regular use of alcohol, is very hard on the liver. Caffeine is hard on the liver, but if it is the only vice a patient has, I allow one cup of coffee per day, and two cups of half decaf. For folks with liver problems, chocolate is very hard on the liver and refined sugars are hard on the liver. Please do not do these things as part of your regular regimen; occasional use is okay. Artificial sweeteners are also very hard on the liver. While we are on the topic of Nutrasweet in particular, many folks ingest Nutrasweet in sodas and carbonated drinks. Carbonated drinks tend to be high in phosphorous which we do not need. We get plenty of phosphorus in other places and too much phosphorus will throw off the calcium balance in our bodies, so please minimize or eliminate the carbonated drinks.

Nutritional Supplements - Getting Your Money's Worth!

Ingredients Without Benefit

Let's move on to nutritional supplementation and how you can tell whether you are getting your money's worth when you buy a product. This requires reading fine print on the labels. The first thing I tell people to watch out for are minerals in forms that are poorly absorbed. Calcium and magnesium take up a lot of space in a product and are the first minerals to check on the label. The more compact forms of calcium are calcium carbonate and calcium phosphate. These are both *very poorly absorbed*. If you read the print on the label and the product says you only need to take one to two pills per day, check the calcium forms because it is probably calcium carbonate or calcium phosphate in this product. (I'll talk about good forms of calcium shortly.)

The next thing to look for are minerals that should not be in any supplement at all. Remember, most of us get plenty of phosphorus in our diet, so if you see phosphorous or phosphate listed on the label, that is a big red flag. We also do not need sodium in a nutritional supplement. If the minerals are in a form, for example, of sodium selenite, that is another red flag for the supplement. The other mineral that we do not need to be getting in supplement form is chloride. For example, some products will contain chloride, like potassium chloride as the potassium source. Between the sodium forms of minerals and the chloride forms of minerals, you are basically getting salt in your nutritional supplement. We certainly don't need to pay for salt in our vitamins!

Perils of Calcium Carbonate

Let's talk about other general problems with supplements. Calcium carbonate is usually extracted from shellfish, and because of lead contamination of the oceans, calcium carbonate is excessively high in lead. This is another reason not to take calcium carbonate. Some of my patients come in and say, "I take Tums for calcium." Antacids like these are calcium carbonate and you are almost certainly getting lead with your calcium if you rely on antacids for calcium. In addition, the reason calcium carbonate is poorly absorbed is because we need an acidic environment in the gastrointestinal tract to absorb calcium properly. Antacids reduce the amount of acid in the stomach, which is the reason we do not absorb calcium very well as calcium carbonate.

Binders and Fillers

Other things to watch for in nutritional supplements are binders and fillers in pills. The pharmaceutical standard for making capsules or tablets allows all kinds of substances to be used as fillers and binders in tablets or capsules, and the manufacturer does not have to tell us that they are are in the product. The FDA does not require these binders and fillers be listed on the label. The best nutritional supplement companies will say what binders and fillers they have included in a product. When you look at a product, check for a place on the label where the manufacturer has listed what other ingredients are in the supplement. A common filler used in the pharmaceutical industry is lactose. This is an obvious problem for people with lactose intolerance. Because the best supplement manufacturers know that you and I care about every ingredient in the products we use, they list binders and fillers on the label. Many will also list whether the product includes other ingredients like dairy, wheat, corn, yeast, soy, etc. An excellent filler is vitamin C. If the label lists any form of vitamin C as a filler, that is likely to be a very good product.

Supplements by Multi-Level Marketing

Another category of things I watch out for is any products being marketed through multi-level marketing. There is a benefit to these programs in that they educate the public about the importance of nutritional supplements. Most of the multi-level marketing products are much more expensive than the same quality supplement from a health food store or from a doctor's office.

One major down side of these products is that many of them contain compounds that are actually toxic. The Blue-Green Algae products have been shown to contain a small amount of toxic species of algae. These can be very dangerous for people with neurological diseases. Blue-Green Algae often contains small levels of toxic metals, things like cadmium or lead as well as toxic chemicals from farm runoff. If you are taking a Blue-Green Algae product (there are some good reasons to take these products) you should be getting an accurate assay from the person you buy it from listing exactly how much of these compounds are present in the product. Another multi-level marketing product that can be a problem is colloidal minerals. Colloidal minerals often have a variety of toxic metals in them including aluminum and lead. In an industrialized society we get plenty of exposure to aluminum and lead. We absorb it from the air we breathe. Please do not take any supplements that contain these toxic metals.

Good Nutritional Supplements

Now that I've talked about things to watch out for, let's talk about the good forms of nutritional supplements. When you are evaluating calcium in a multiple, look for calcium citrate, or calcium citrate-malate. Of the chelated forms of calcium, these have been shown to have the best absorption. Magnesium is fairly easily absorbed, and many forms of magnesium are good. Better forms of magnesium will be magnesium citrate and magnesium glycinate. Some manufacturers will chelate calcium and magnesium with rice bran or rice protein. This is also a good form of these minerals.

In order for us to get good absorption of minerals, they need to be combined in a chelated form. Chelated forms include aspartate, picolinate, or glycinate; these are all good forms of minerals. Chromium can be GTF, which stands for "glucose tolerance factor". When you look at the label you will see, for example, copper as copper glycinate or copper aspartate, or zinc as zinc picolinate. If a product does not tell you what form they have combined the minerals with, be suspicious.

Vitamin E occurs as either d-alpha tocopherol or dl-alpha-tocopherol. Chemically, vitamin E is both forms, but our body cannot use vitamin E as l-alpha tocopherol. If you buy the synthetic mixture dl-alpha tocopherol, you are wasting your money and your time. The two forms that I have people look for on the label are either "d-alpha tocopherol" or "mixed natural tocopherols." These can be used as vitamin E by our bodies.

Another sign of a good quality product is the forms the B vitamins are in. A good quality multiple or B-complex supplement will have some of the B vitamins in activated forms. Activated forms of the B vitamins are ready for our cells and liver to use without being transformed. When folks have sluggish liver function they respond much better to activated B vitamins. For example: B6 is pyridoxine and activated B6 is pyridoxal 5' phosphate or P5P. Riboflavin is B2 and activated riboflavin is riboflavin 5' phosphate.

If you check the label and a product has the calcium in a good form and some activated B vitamins you can be fairly confident that the manufacturer has gone to a good deal of trouble to exceed the FDA requirements and provide you with a quality nutritional supplement.

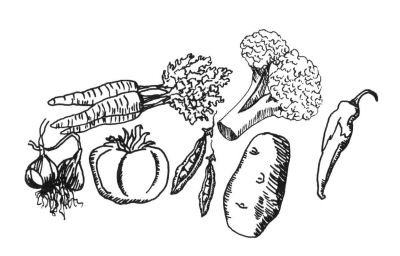

Chapter 4
Demystifying Diets

Hello and welcome to Tape Four of the Free to Be Well© series. On this tape I will be talking about food and diet. I would like to say first that, as a clinician, I am always very hesitant to talk to people about how to eat because most of us have foods that we like and ways that we like to eat. It is a fairly personal thing to be sitting in my chair and making suggestions or recommendations to my patients about how to eat. Please remember that whatever I say on this tape, take what makes sense to you. Hopefully I can persuade you about eliminating toxic things from your diet. But other than that, how you eat is really up to you. You need to make sure you are comfortable with whatever diet you chose to follow. I am not talking about weight-loss diets, I am just talking about the foods you chose to eat and the foods you chose not to eat. Feeling good about food does not just mean feeling good on the diet, it also means that emotionally you are comfortable with the foods you are eating.

Weight Loss Diets

Before I get into specific diets, I want to talk about weight-loss diets. There is a lot of money to be made in this country with weight-loss diets and the weight-loss industry in general. We are bombarded with lots of marketing by the weight-loss industry. Many diet books you see on the bookstore shelf have either a primary or a secondary slant on weight-loss. When you look at the front cover, one of the big things they are using to sell the book is that you will lose weight if you do whatever their program is. Many of the diets I will be talking about on this tape have been promoted as weight-loss diets in order to sell the books, but that is not the primary purpose of the diet. This does not mean that you will *not* lose weight on any of the diets, but it also does not mean that you *will* lose weight on any of the diets.

Getting back to weight loss diets, whether you are large or small, long-term low-calorie dieting is very unhealthy for your body for several reasons. It puts the body into a starvation state in which the body starts using proteins as an energy source. Using protein as an energy source means the body is eating up muscle tissue. This is not just skeletal muscle or the voluntary muscles that we use to do things, but also our heart muscle. Burning protein for energy is extremely hard on the kidneys because it increases the protein byproducts that the kidneys need to eliminate in the urine. Starvation diets are toxic to the liver. As we learned on Tape Three, liver health is extremely important to the health of the rest of our body. In addition to a low-calorie diet causing destruction of heart muscle, it is also destructive to the blood vessel linings. The metabolic products that get released when we go on a low-calorie diet actually accelerate the inflammation we talked about on Tape One that causes atherosclerosis.

The Truth about Being Large

What all this means to me as a clinician is that I would much prefer to see my larger patients stay large, than lose weight, gain weight, and lose weight with low-calorie diets. This cycle of weight loss and gain and loss is destructive to the heart and blood vessel linings and contributes significantly to heart disease and atherosclerosis. I know this contradicts a lot of what you have been told, that people who are overweight, large, or fat (whatever you want to call these folks) will tend to have heart attacks, high blood pressure, diabetes and all the rest of it.

I would like to present another theory about why folks who are large or fat in North America tend to have these kinds of problems. It has been shown in studies that heart disease and high blood pressure are diseases of stress. If we look at the data from another point of view, we see that people who are large in this culture are under a lot of stress because of how they are treated by those who are not large. There is a general expectation in this culture that in order to be beautiful, we have to be thin. I would propose that maybe the increased incidence of high blood pressure and heart disease in people who are large in North America has more to do with the stress they are under because of the expectations of society and because of the way they are treated on a daily basis than it has to do with the fact that they are large.

Remember the cycle of long-term, low-calorie diets with weight loss, weight gain, and weight loss is destructive to blood vessels and to the heart. Effects of dieting will also cause high blood pressure and heart disease. We have no proof in North America that the increased incidence of heart disease and high blood pressure in this population is due to being large rather than the effects of dieting. The health problems that we associate with folks being large may really be due to diets. Another important point is that in countries where large folks are considered beautiful, there is no greater incidence of heart disease and high blood pressure in folks that are fat versus folks that are thin. Stated another way, in countries where large folks are considered beautiful, both thin people and fat people have the *same rate* of heart disease and high blood pressure.

Benefits of Being Large

There are diseases that being fat protects us from. One is osteoporosis. Men and women who are large have a much lower risk of osteoporosis. Because bone responds to the forces placed on it and the more weight bearing we do with our bones, the more dense they will become. Weight bearing exercise helps prevent osteoporosis, but being heavy also helps prevent osteoporosis because more is demanded of the bones in terms of weight bearing. For women during menopause, being large also helps diminish menopausal symptoms. The reason for this is that estrogen is also made by body fat. Carrying an extra 10-20 lbs. of body fat actually helps diminish the discomfort associated with menopause because women are getting estrogen from the body fat they are carrying. Some sources are actually recommending that women approaching menopause should be 10-20 lbs. heavier than is generally recommended to help them be more comfortable and actually healthier long term through their menopausal years.

Diet Summaries

Let's move on to talking about the various diets. I'm going to summarize each of these diets. It is not possible on a one-hour tape to do justice to the diets that I have chosen to summarize. Most of these diets have several books you can read about them if you want to delve into any one of them in detail. I am going to list representative titles and authors. Each of these diets has a different paradigm about what makes our bodies sick and how our bodies can get well through food. For you, as the audience and the person choosing how you want to eat, the decision about what diet to follow or whether to follow a combination of two or more diets is a personal decision based on your body, how you feel, your lifestyle, your ability to cook things at home, or the things you can find if you need to eat out. The bottom line is: you are the one who has the decision-making power and the responsibility to chose what you are going to eat. I strongly recommend if any of these diets appeal to you, that you get a book about the diet and read it before you decide to change how you eat.

Fit for Life

The first diet I am going to talk about is popularly known as the Fit for Life Diet. This is based on the Natural Hygiene movement that started in the United States in the mid 1800's. This system teaches that disease can be cured through diet. The most popular book on the subject is *Fit for Life* by Harvey and Marilyn Diamond. The Fit for Life Diet is based mainly on fresh fruits and vegetables and uses the principles of food combining. According to this philosophy, the day is broken up into three portions; from noon to 8 p.m. is for eating and digestion, from 8 p.m. to 4 a.m. is for absorption and use of nutrients, and from 4 a.m. to noon is for elimination of body waste and food debris. A central principle of this diet is adequately facilitating elimination of toxins from the body. One way that toxins are produced in the body is through cellular metabolism and death of old cells. Another way toxins are produced in the body is through inefficient digestion and assimilation, leaving byproducts of undigested food in the gut. The body has four organs of elimination, the bowel, bladder, lungs, and skin.

The elimination of toxins is facilitated by eating a diet of living foods. This means fresh fruits and vegetables, and high water content foods. Therefore, 70% of the diet is based on fresh fruits and vegetables and only 30% of the diet is what are called concentrated foods. Concentrated foods are everything else except fruits and vegetables. Grains, meats, dairy products, etc., should be kept to only 30% of the diet. In addition to the high water content in fresh fruits and vegetables, fruits and vegetables are also high in enzymes. This means they are living foods. When we cook fruits and vegetables, we destroy the enzymes in them. Additionally, in order to facilitate enzymes working properly to digest our food we should not drink water with our meals. Then our own digestive enzymes and the enzymes in the fruits and vegetables we eat will work together to aid digestion.

Food combining is based on the theory that our stomach and small intestines cannot handle more than one type of food at a time. For example, we should never eat fruit with any other type of food. With food combining, we should not combine more than one type of the concentrated foods at a time. So if we are eating meat, we can have vegetables raw or lightly steamed, but not potatoes or bread with meat. Conversely, if we are having pasta or bread, we can have these with vegetables, but not with meat or dairy. According to this philosophy, isolation of foods from each other (i.e. not having grains or potatoes together, not having grains or meats together) facilitates the ability of the body to digest them properly and thus facilitates the ability of the body to eliminate waste products properly.

Fruit is rich in nutrients and requires less energy to be digested than any other food. Because fruit is so easy to digest and it can ferment so easily in the gastro-intestinal tract, it should always be eaten on an empty stomach and never eaten with any other type of food. On the Fit for Life Diet only fruit is eaten until noon. From the time you wake up until noon, the only foods eaten are fresh fruit and fruit juice. This facilitates the body's normal cycle of elimination which, remember, goes from 4 a.m. to noon. Because fruit is so easily digested, it facilitates the body's ability to eliminate wastes. The second cycle, from noon to 8 p.m., is appropriation, or eating and digestion. This is the time to eat meals with other foods. This is the time to eat meals with the concentrated foods, the non-fruits and non-vegetables, and also the time to eat vegetables. Digesting these foods takes more energy, hence the reason they should be properly combined to minimize the energy used in digesting the foods. The assimilation cycle, from 8 p.m. to 4 a.m., of absorption and use of foods, is a time not to eat but to give the body a chance to absorb and use the nutrients in the food you have consumed during the day. Ceasing eating before 8 p.m. also gives a chance for the food to be done in the stomach before we go to bed at night. This diet discourages the use of meat, eggs, and dairy products.

In their book Harvey and Marilyn Diamond discuss the same topics I have talked about previously on these tapes. These are the problems with antibiotics that are fed to animals prior to slaughter, arsenic that is fed to chickens to prevent parasites and stimulate egg production, and antibiotics and hormones that are fed to dairy cows. They recommend that if you are going to get meat, to get free-range and organically raised meat, and for dairy and eggs to get organically produced products and limit these foods to one meal per day. Again, because of combining rules, you would only have one of these foods each day at one meal.

The main principles of this diet are that 70% of the foods you eat are to be high water content foods (fresh fruits and vegetables) and prior to noon eat only fresh fruits and fruit juices.

Macrobiotic Principle

The next diet I will discuss is the Macrobiotic Diet. The main sources of macrobiotic information in this country are Michio Kushi and George Ohsawa. There are a variety of macrobiotic books. The book I have used for reference is *The Macrobiotic Way* by Michio Kushi. Macrobiotic diets are based on bringing humans closer to the natural world and preventing sickness and unhappiness by adopting a diet and a way of life that brings us into harmony with our environment.

A Macrobiotic Overview

Macrobiotic diets emphasize the use of whole grains and locally produced foods. In other words, we should eat fruits and vegetables that grow in our local region at the time when they are in season. A macrobiotic diet is based on 50-60% whole grain products, 20-30% locally grown, preferably organically grown vegetables, 5-10% beans and sea vegetables (i.e. seaweed), 5-10% soups, and 5% condiments and other foods like beverages, fish, and desserts. Therefore, 70-90% of the food consumed on a macrobiotic diet would be whole grains, whole grain products, and fruits and vegetables. Macrobiotic diets are mainly vegetarian, relying for protein on soy-based foods like tofu and tempeh, seitan which is made from wheat and is high in protein, and amasake which is a milk-like drink made from brown rice or almonds. Small amounts of white-meat fish are allowed and certain shell fish.

Whole Grains in the Macrobiotic Diet

The cornerstone of the macrobiotic diet is whole grains. These give the body an even, long-lasting source of carbohydrates for energy. Complex carbohydrates burn clean. In other words, they break down into water and carbon dioxide which are easily eliminated. They also produce glucose that the body uses for energy. Complex carbohydrates do not cause the insulin swings that refined sugars do, and they do not leave behind waste products that are difficult for the body to eliminate. Protein sources on a macrobiotic diet are from whole grains, beans, especially soy foods, vegetables, sea vegetables, seeds, and white-meat fish. Red meat, poultry, and dairy products are not allowed on a macrobiotic diet. Excessive protein in the diet causes build up of toxic compounds in the body, urea and uric acid, also excess fat and cholesterol that the body needs to eliminate. These compounds building up in the blood can cause depletion of minerals from the body. A high-protein diet can increase the risk of cancer.

Fiber and Fat in the Macrobiotic Diet

Fat in the macrobiotic diet comes from oils that occur naturally in whole foods. Small amounts of oil are also used in cooking. Acceptable oils in macrobiotic cooking are unrefined, which preserves the naturally occurring vitamin E in the oil and prevents oil from becoming rancid. The mix of foods in a macrobiotic diet along with the high fiber of the diet promote the health of the small and large intestines and also improves the ecology of the mix of microflora in the large intestine. Foods that promote the health of the large intestine are whole grains, beans, and vegetables that are rich in fiber and fermented foods used in the macrobiotic diet. Macrobiotic fermented foods are things like miso, tempeh, tamari, umeboshi, sauerkraut, and pickles. These specialized fermented foods help promote the growth of beneficial bacteria in the large intestine by producing lactic acid.

Macrobiotic Greens and Grains

A macrobiotic diet includes a wide variety of fresh vegetables and leafy greens including dandelion greens, parsley, and sea vegetables. A macrobiotic diet also includes fruits. Macrobiotic diets eaten properly are extremely rich in vitamins and minerals. In this philosophy, foods should be eaten as close to their natural state as possible. For example, grains we should consume are whole barley, whole corn, brown rice, or whole oats as opposed to grains that have been made into pasta, cracked, corn grits, or rice cakes where the foods have been pre-processed before we eat them. Grains to avoid are: white flour products, refined grain cereals, breads, crackers, or cakes made with yeast, and baked goods that contain eggs or dairy products.

Macrobiotic Vegetables

The vegetable families are divided into green and leafy vegetables that grow above ground, vegetables that grow on the ground (like squashes), and vegetables that grow under the ground like carrots and potatoes. Vegetables that are preferred on a macrobiotic diet are: the entire cabbage family, carrot tops, most of the squashes, dark green leafy vegetables with the exception of spinach. Preferred greens include things like chives, collard greens, dandelion greens, mustard greens, scallions, radish greens, parsley, and watercress. Root vegetables are things like radishes, onions, dandelion roots, carrots, burdock root, parsnips, and turnips. Vegetables to avoid include all of the nightshade family. Potatoes, tomatoes, eggplant, and bell peppers   are members of the nightshade family. Green and red peppers are avoided on a macrobiotic diet. There are a variety of sea vegetables that are used in a macrobiotic diet. To use these properly, I strongly recommend getting a macrobiotic cook book. Recommended beans on a macrobiotic diet include aduki beans, chick peas, lentils, miso, tempeh, tofu, and nato (or fermented soy beans).

Macrobiotic Condiments

There are also a wide variety of condiments and seasonings that are allowed on a macrobiotic diet. They tend to be simply produced things like ginger, gomashio (which is a mixture of sea salt and ground sesame seeds), grated diakon radish, seaweed condiment, pickled vegetables and sauerkraut, onions, scallions, parsley, sea salt, tamari (a wheat-free soy sauce), and horseradish. Things that are not allowed in the condiment category on a macrobiotic diet are things like mayonnaise, margarine, commercial soy sauce, most vinegars, many types of spices, and any artificially or chemically processed seasoning product.

Macrobiotic Sweets and Beverages

Natural sweeteners are allowed occasionally. A macrobiotic diet really relies on the natural flavor of whole fresh foods. Fresh and dried fruits, especially local fruits that are organically raised, are allowed for occasional use in a macrobiotic diet. For those of us who live in temperate climates, including North America, tropical fruits should not be consumed. Local, organically raised fruits, either fresh or dried, can be used in moderation and should be cooked. A macrobiotic diet does not allow most of the common drinks used by North Americans, including black tea, coffee, alcoholic drinks, milk, and orange juice. Colas and carbonated drinks are also not allowed on a macrobiotic diet. The macrobiotic diet relies on a variety of natural teas, bancha tea, roasted barley tea, or roasted rice tea. Spring or well water and amasake are allowed as beverages. As with the Fit for Life Diet, on a macrobiotic diet you do not drink water with your meal. There are other herbal teas allowed and occasional fruit juices are allowed.

The Yin and Yang of the Macrobiotic Diet

Another basic principle of the macrobiotic diet is balancing yin and yang. These are the two opposing energies of the universe. Trying to explain the philosophy of yin and yang on a tape of this length is far beyond the scope of this project. However, a central principle of macrobiotic eating is balancing the yin and yang energies of the foods. Macrobiotic diets applied properly for people with diseases can be extremely beneficial. To use a macrobiotic diet to heal disease, the diet should be prescribed by a health care practitioner who is knowledgeable in the use of macrobiotic diets. For people who are basically healthy, the macrobiotic diet can be extremely beneficial in that it advocates the use of whole grains, and whole foods closest to their natural state. This eliminates many of the chemicals and contaminants we are generally exposed to in the Standard American Diet (SAD).

The Anti-Candida Diet

The next diet on our list is the Anti-Candida Diet. There are many good books on this topic. My source on this diet is *The Yeast Connection* by William G. Crook, M.D. The goal of this diet is to fight candida infections and/or prevent recurrence of candida problems. Systemic candida infections can cause a multitude of health problems including joint pain, headaches, fatigue, indigestion, athlete's foot, or chronic vaginal yeast infections.

Foods to Eliminate

The candida diet eliminates all foods that would facilitate the growth of yeast. This includes alcohol, sugars, concentrated sweeteners, breads that are yeast risen, and fruit juices. A more detailed list of foods that you must avoid on a candida diet are any foods containing sugars including honey, molasses, maple syrup, and maple sugar. All packaged and processed foods must be eliminated because they often have sugar added to them. Foods containing yeast and mold should also be eliminated. These include cheeses, alcoholic beverages, breads and pastries, condiments, sauces, and vinegar-containing foods, smoked meats, edible fungi such as mushrooms, malt products, melon, coffee and tea, fruit juice, dried and candied fruit, and any leftovers. Anything kept in your refrigerator more than three days has mold growing on it.

Foods to Consume with Caution

Foods you can eat on a candida diet with caution are the high carbohydrate vegetables, or starchy vegetables. These are things like sweet potatoes, red potatoes, corn, parsnips, peas and beans, and whole grains like barley, corn, millet, oats, rice, and wheat. Bread and biscuits can be eaten with caution on a candida diet as long as they are not yeast risen and as long as they are not leftover.

Foods to Eat Freely

Foods that can be eaten freely on a candida diet include non-starchy vegetables, soy bean products, meats, fish, poultry, and eggs. Seeds, nuts, and oils are allowed. Nuts and seeds need to be either dry roasted or unprocessed and oils need to be unrefined. A caution regarding nuts; many people are sensitive to nuts. If they cause you symptoms, they are not allowed on the candida diet.

Making Personal Adjustments in the Diet

This rigid diet needs to be adhered to for several weeks. After that time you can experiment with a few foods. These include all fresh vegetables (you would be allowed to have starchy vegetables), all fresh fruits, all grains. Fish, meat, eggs, nuts, seeds, and oils continue to be allowed. You can experiment with adding back some of the foods that contain yeast, but if they aggravate your system, then you have to leave them out. You must continue to avoid any foods containing sugars, sweeteners, and refined sugars. For the typical person with candida, the diet alone is not going to be sufficient treatment, so you need to seek the help of a qualified practitioner. Also, please note that the candida diet varies quite a bit from the first two diets we talked about on this tape. This diet allows much more protein, especially animal-based protein than either the macrobiotic diet or the Fit for Life Diet.

The Four-Day Rotation Diet

Another part of the candida diet is the four-day rotation diet. This diet is used for people with food allergies and for people with candida. The immune system takes four days to fully complete its reaction to foods. On a rotation diet you could have any specific type of food only one day in every four. On day one you might have corn and different dairy products and day two you might choose wheat and egg products, and the third day you could have barley and soy products, and the fourth day you might have rice and chicken. This is a representative example. In the four days, you would not have more than one day when you ate the same food. Rotation diets tend to be extremely complicated. The best reference I am familiar with is Sally Rockwell. She has many resources about rotation diets for both food allergies and candida. [ed. note: see resource list]

Vegan Diets

The next diet I would like to talk to you about is the Vegan Diet. My resource for this is *The New Farm Vegetarian Cookbook*. Vegan diets are completely free of any animal foods. They are vegetarian without dairy, eggs, fish, or poultry. A vegan diet allows processed foods as long as they are free of animal products and is based on the avoidance of cruelty to animals rather than a specific approach to health care and prevention of disease. However, there is a lot of data to support the fact that vegetarians are, by and large, healthier than people who eat animal products regularly.

For those of you who have a hard time conceiving of a diet that is free of eggs, dairy, fish, and meat, there are some very tasty recipes in this cookbook including French toast with no eggs and no milk. There is also an excellent gravy recipe. These diets rely mainly on grains, whole grains, soy products, vegetables and fruits. Nutritional yeast is a versatile component of these diets. Nutritional yeast is high in B vitamins and protein.

The McDougall Program

You may have heard of the Dean Ornish or John McDougall programs. Both Dean Ornish and John McDougall are medical doctors. The resource book I am using is *The McDougall Program* by John McDougall, M.D.

Dr. McDougall found by studying the published scientific literature that many of the diseases we see in Western Culture are related to our diet. These include cancers, many diseases of the digestive system and colon, high blood pressure and heart attacks, and kidney diseases. For arthritis, high blood pressure, kidney diseases and gastrointestinal diseases, the best treatment is a change in diet. In summary, the McDougall Program involves a diet centered around carbohydrates, fruits, and vegetables and the elimination of foods containing protein and fat. It allows no meat, dairy products, poultry, fish, eggs, oils, and even vegetarian foods rich in fat are limited. The program includes moderate exercise on a daily basis.

Checking your Statistics

Dr. McDougall is an advocate of collecting statistics on yourself when you start the program and when you finish the 12-day section of the program. Things he encourages discovering are your weight, blood pressure, and your cholesterol, triglycerides (the fat in your blood), glucose (the sugar in your blood), and uric acid, all before and after the

12-day program. You certainly can do the McDougall program without getting these statistics though.

McDougall's Good Foods

The cornerstone of the McDougall program are what he calls the starch staples. These are whole grains, whole grain flours, whole grain egg-free pastas, oriental noodles, roots (like burdock, sweet potatoes, tapioca, white potatoes, yams, and jicama), winter squashes (like butternut, acorn, and buttercup), and beans (including peas, lentils, and all varieties of dried beans). On the McDougall program, however, soy beans are too high in fat to be allowed as a staple food.

Other foods to eat liberally on the McDougall diet are fresh and frozen vegetables and fruits. Packaged foods are allowed on the McDougall diet; processed foods are not. Salt and sugar in packaged foods are not allowed. Oils and fats in packaged foods are not allowed. Sulphur dioxide and MSG are not allowed on this diet. When reading the label on packaged foods, you need to really read carefully. Sugars can be maltose, sucrose, dextrose, fructose, and corn syrup which all are hidden in foods. When buying cereals, breads, pastas, rice cakes, etc., labels should be examined carefully for alien ingredients or chemical ingredients. McDougall has a list in his book of acceptable brands of packaged foods including cereals, breads, crackers, soups, pastas, mixes, salad dressing, and a variety of condiments. The McDougall Diet is similar to a Vegan Diet with the additional restriction of fats and protein.

The Zone Diet

The next diet I will discuss is the Zone Diet which, as you will see, is very different from the McDougall diet. There are two or three books about this diet by Barry Sears, *The Zone* and *Mastering The Zone*. A similar book by a husband and wife who are medical doctors, Michael Eades and Mary Dan Eades, is called _Protein Power_. The Zone Diet is aimed at managing insulin and glucagon levels by diet. Insulin is a hormone that moves sugar into cells and lowers blood sugar when it gets high. Glucagon is responsible for raising blood sugar when it gets low. Insulin converts glucose and protein to fat. It also promotes storage of fat in fat cells, increases the body's production of cholesterol, and promotes fluid retention by the kidneys. Glucagon, in addition to raising blood sugar when it gets low, decreases the body's cholesterol levels, releases fat from fat cells, and promotes the use of fats and protein as an energy source. Glucagon also promotes the release of excess fluid by the kidneys.

The Influence of Carbohydrates

The types of foods we have in a meal will influence the release of these hormones. Carbohydrates raise insulin the most. The greatest increase in insulin levels happens with a meal that is high in carbohydrates _and_ low in protein. On the other hand, protein stimulates glucagon which will in turn reduce insulin. Fats are neutral as far as insulin and glucagon are concerned.

The cornerstone of the Zone Diet is to balance the intake of protein and carbohydrates at every meal. This balances insulin and glucagon levels. Fat is used to slow down the entry of carbohydrates from the gut into the blood stream and also to cause release of a hormone from the stomach that sends a message to the brain to say stop eating.

A zone diet divides carbohydrates into favorable and unfavorable carbohydrates. Carbohydrates vary in their ability to cause the body to produce insulin. This is called the glycemic index. Some carbohydrates have a high glycemic index, meaning they cause the blood sugar to go up a lot, and insulin levels will also go up. Other carbohydrates have a low glycemic index which means they will not raise blood sugar levels much and will not promote much insulin release. On the Zone Diet favorable carbohydrates are fruits and vegetables. Unfavorable carbohydrates are starches like potatoes and grains like cereals, pastas, and breads. Processed starches have a higher glycemic index than whole foods, for example the glycemic index of instant potatoes is much higher than a baked potato. This is because the sugars and starches in the instant potatoes get released into the blood stream more quickly as the potato cell walls are destroyed in the instant potatoes.

Balancing Essential Fatty Acids

The Zone Diet also recommends balancing essential fatty acids to avoid inflammation in the body. Fatty red meats, egg yolks, and organ meats are kept to a minimum because they are high in arachidonic acid which promotes inflammation. Since the omega 6 fatty acids are included in the proteins in the Zone Diet, additional sources are limited. These generally come from oils such as sunflower, safflower, and soybean oil, so these oils should be avoided. Omega 3 fatty acids are encouraged and these are present in fish. Fins and scales type fish, especially salmon, are a good source of omega 3 fatty acids. Monounsaturated fats are hormone neutral and are promoted as a source of dietary fat on the Zone Diet. Sources of monounsaturated fats include nuts, avocados, and olives.

Food Blocks

The Zone Diet looks at foods in terms of blocks. Protein blocks contain 7 grams of protein. Carbohydrate blocks contain 9 grams of insulin promoting carbohydrates. At every meal for every protein block you consume you need to consume one carbohydrate block. Fat blocks on the Zone Diet contain 1½ gm of fat which is the equivalent of ⅓ teaspoon of olive oil. At every meal for every protein block and carbohydrate block, one fat block should be included. In addition to types of foods eaten at a meal, timing is important on the Zone Diet. You shouldn't go more than five hours between meals, and for most folks that means five meals per day. This is usually done as three meals and two snacks.

To give you an idea of the portions of blocks, one block of protein is equivalent to 1 oz. of meat, poultry, or fish, 1 oz. of most cheeses, and 3 oz. of tofu. The amount of carbohydrate in your carbohydrate blocks varies depending on the type of vegetable or fruit. Some typical examples of one block of favorable carbohydrate are: a half cup of salsa, half an apple, a whole peach, half an orange, 1½ cups of broccoli, one medium artichoke, 1 cup of cooked green or wax beans, 3 cups cooked bok choy, 1½ cups cooked zucchini, 4 cups of lettuce, or 2 tomatoes. Examples of one block of unfavorable carbohydrates are: ¼ of a small bagel, ¼ cup cooked pasta, ⅓ cup cooked potato, a 1 inch square of cornbread, ½ slice of whole grain bread, or 1/5 cup rice, either brown or white. Fat blocks include ⅓ teaspoon almond butter, ⅓ teaspoon of olive oil, 1 tablespoon of guacamole, three olives, or six peanuts.

If you chose to follow the Zone Diet, I recommend getting a copy of one of the books I have mentioned. I would like to add a cautionary note here. I *do not recommend* the Zone Diet for people with kidney problems, diabetes, or those over 60. If any of these apply to you or you have any serious medical condition like heart disease or high blood pressure, *do not* go on this diet without consulting a qualified health care practitioner.

Blood Type Diets

These are diets based on our blood type which is genetically inherited. My reference for this is *Eat Right For Your Type* by Dr. Peter J. D'Adamo. We each have antibodies in our blood because of our blood type. These antibodies are programmed to seek out and destroy proteins of specific shapes that are present in other blood types. Foods that we eat also have their unique proteins, and for each blood type there are foods with protein shapes that will activate the antibodies in our blood to go on a seek and destroy mission. The end result of this is irritation and cell damage. Foods that will cause these reactions are different for each of the different blood types. The most common blood types are blood type O and blood type A. Other blood types are blood type B and blood type AB.

Blood Type O

Folks with different blood types also have different variations on the digestive system. For example, type O folks tend to have more stomach acid then type A folks. Type O folks do not do well on dairy products and grains. Wheat gluten is particularly irritating for the type O digestive tract. Type O's tend to do well with lean red meats, poultry, and fish. Remember, meats in your diet should be free-range, grass-fed meats and free-range poultry. Type O's also do well on most kinds of fish but should curtail or eliminate dairy products. Type O's should eliminate wheat. Acceptable grains for type O include amaranth, rice, buckwheat, barley, and millet. Quinoa, rye, and spelt are also acceptable for type O's. Most varieties of beans are acceptable for type O's except lentils, kidney beans, and navy beans; however, type O's should eat all beans in moderation. Type O's should get carbohydrates from vegetables and fruits rather than pasta, grains, and beans. Dried fruits are a good snack food rather than chips or crackers. Type O's should also avoid condiments and caffeinated beverages like coffee.

Blood Type A

As opposed to type O's, type A's tend to do well on vegetarian diets. Type A's should refrain from all red meat. Poultry is acceptable in moderation for type A's. Many types of fish are okay for type A. However, shell fish and other non-kosher type fishes are not. Examples of shellfish are clam, crab, oysters, octopus, eel, crayfish, lobster, mussels, scallops, shrimp, and squid. Type A's tolerate dairy products better than type O's do, however, they should moderate their dairy products. Dairy products that are acceptable to type A's include yogurt, goat cheeses, farmer's cheese, feta cheese, mozzarella, ricotta, and kefir. As opposed to type O's who should not have peanuts, type A's do well on peanuts. Type A's also do well on a variety of nuts, but should avoid Brazil nuts, cashews, and pistachios. Type A's do well on the proteins found in beans and they also tolerate most cereals and grains well. However, many type A's do not tolerate wheat very well. As far as vegetables, type A's do not tolerate the nightshade vegetables well: eggplant, potatoes, tomatoes, and yams. Type A's should not eat peppers of any variety. Type A's should eat fruit frequently and most fruits are fine for type A's except bananas, plantains, melons, mangos, and oranges. Type A's do well with coffee, either decaf or regular, but should avoid black tea and soda.

Blood Type B

Type B's tend to have flexible dietary choices, but they do have some foods they need to avoid. Chicken can be a major problem for type B's and should definitely be avoided. To some type B's, beef is a problem. The recommended meats for type B's are mutton, lamb, rabbit, and venison. Turkey is acceptable for type B's and pork is not. There are many fishes that are acceptable for type B's, however, the same shell fish that are unacceptable for type A's are unacceptable for type B's. Regarding dairy products, type B's are the only blood type that can consume diary products liberally. However, a small minority of type B's may have a lactose intolerance which is not an immune problem. In the event of lactose intolerance, cultured dairy products, in which the lactose has been predigested, should be used. These are yogurt, kefir, or cheeses. In general, type B's do not do well with nuts. Some acceptable nuts for type B's are almonds, Brazil nuts, chestnuts, macadamias, pecans, and walnuts. For type B's cashews, filberts, peanuts, pistachios, sunflower seeds, and sesame seeds should be avoided. On the bean front, type B's should avoid garbanzo beans, pinto beans, lentils, and black beans. Oats, rice, and quinoa are acceptable grains for type B's. Most type B's do not tolerate wheat very well. Type B's should also avoid barley, corn, and rye. Among the vegetables, type B's should avoid artichokes, avocados, corn, olives, mung sprouts, and tomatoes. However, among the nightshades type B's can have eggplant, potatoes, peppers, and yams. Type B's should also eat fruit liberally. Type B's handle condiments generally better than type O or type A, but should avoid catsup. Type B's can have coffee and tea and should not have soda of any type.

Blood Type AB

Type AB's are a combination of blood type A and blood type B in terms of the foods that are well tolerated or the foods that are not tolerated. Type AB's should not have beef, pork, or chicken. Beneficial meats for type AB's are lamb, mutton, rabbit, and turkey. Type AB's tend to tolerate dairy foods well, especially those that have been cultured like yogurt or kefir. Type AB's can have peanuts, walnuts, and chestnuts, but should avoid filberts, poppy seeds, sesame seeds, and sunflower seeds. Lentils and soy beans are good for type AB; however, garbanzos, black beans, kidney beans, and lima beans are not. Most AB's seem to tolerate wheat in limited amounts. Corn and buckwheat should be avoided by AB's. Among the vegetables, AB's seem to tolerate the nightshades adequately. They should avoid artichokes, avocados, corn, and all kinds of peppers. Type AB's should avoid pickled condiments and catsup. Coffee is acceptable for type AB, but soda and black tea are not.

Considering the Blood Type Diet

If the elements of this diet captivate your curiosity, I would strongly recommend you look for a book about blood type diets as the lists I have given are not complete by any means. Because of the different digestive tracts of the different blood types, the relatively higher protein content of the Zone diet tends to work well for blood type O and blood type B. However, if you are blood type A, you probably will not feel very well on the Zone Diet. Conversely, the higher vegetarian content of a diet like the McDougall Diet or the Fit for Life Diet is likely to work better for type A's.

The Phytonutrient Diet, aka the Detoxification Diet

The next diet I would like to discuss is my favorite among the detox diets, also known as the phytonutrient diet. My source book for this is *The Twenty Day Rejuvenation Diet Program* by Jeffrey Bland, Ph.D. This Detoxification Diet is founded on research worldwide documenting how food affects our physiology. Dr. Bland has a unique ability to collect and synthesize volumes of scientific data into a clinically useable whole. The goal of this diet is really three-fold. First is to eliminate all foods that are either difficult to digest or metabolize or likely to cause food sensitivities or allergies. Second is to introduce foods, especially nutrients from plants that help heal up the digestive tract. Third is to introduce specific nutritious foods, especially from plants, that help improve the liver's ability to get rid of toxic substances, both the toxins that come from outside our body and the toxins that are made inside our body.

Foods to Avoid

Of the foods that are eliminated on this diet, the first group is foods that contain gluten, including: wheat, barley, oats, rye, triticale, spelt, and kamut. Of course for most of us, the gluten containing food we eat most frequently is wheat. Other foods that are not allowed on the phytonutrient diet are milk, diary products, and eggs. Beverages that are not allowed are all alcoholic beverages and all beverages containing caffeine. Soft drinks are not allowed. Salty foods, sugars, and foods high in fats are not allowed on the phytonutrient diet. Foods containing chemical flavorings, colorings, preservatives, or artificial sweeteners are not allowed.

Foods to Include

Grains that are allowed on the phytonutrient diet are rice, corn, buckwheat, millet, tapioca, amaranth, and quinoa. Packaged foods are allowed on this diet as long as they do not include artificial sweeteners, sugars, salt, or other chemical ingredients.

All manner of organic fruits and vegetables are allowed on this diet with the exception of avocado which may be eaten in small amounts and coconut. Nuts are allowed in moderation. Unsweetened fruit juice and dried fruit are allowed. For beverages water, mineral water, sodium free seltzer, and herb teas are allowed.

This diet also has a list of must-eat foods. These are things you must eat every day. The must-eat foods include foods high in carotene and foods high in vitamin C. Carotene containing foods are any of your orange-yellow vegetables or fruits. Vitamin C containing foods are citrus fruits, broccoli, strawberries, tomatoes, melons, potatoes, bell peppers, Brussels sprouts, and cabbage. Fresh pure water, eight 8 oz. glasses per day is also a must on this diet. An antioxidant vitamin supplement as well as a multi-vitamin and mineral supplement is important.

Plant foods important on the phytonutrient diet include the cruciferous vegetables like broccoli, cauliflower, cabbage, and Brussels sprouts; soy foods, especially tofu; and vegetables that include carotenoid compounds. Carotenoid containing foods are dark, green, leafy vegetables and red or orange fruits and vegetables. Citrus fruits are valuable for their bioflavonoid compounds, and garlic and onions are valuable for their sulphur-containing compounds. Many of these beneficial compounds in fruits and vegetables are only available if the fruits and vegetables are eaten fresh, lightly steamed, or juiced. Long cooking or canning destroys many of the valuable compounds in these foods.

The phytonutrient diet also emphasizes carbohydrates that have a low glycemic index. This means they will facilitate good blood sugar control. The grain with the lowest glycemic index is barley. Various beans or legumes also tend to have very low glycemic indices, and are good sources of carbohydrates that do not raise blood sugar. The phytonutrient diet is rich in both soluble and insoluble fiber.

Dr. Bland's book has lots of recipes and ideas how to use this diet. When I put my patients on this diet, I give them an exchange list and tell them I want them eating about 4 oz. of protein per day. A good protein source is fish or poultry. If the protein source is legumes or soy, they are allowed more. I recommend a minimum of two cups vegetables per day and the equivalent of about two cups of fruit per day. Total fat for the day would be the equivalent of about 4 teaspoons of olive oil. They are allowed twelve servings of starch. A starch serving is one slice of rice bread, half a cup of rice pasta, or ¾ cup of Rice Chex.

A Scientific Connection Between Diet and Health

Aside from the diet information in Dr. Bland's book, I encourage many of my patients to read it because it explains so much of the recent research regarding health, disease, and why we tend to get sick in western cultures. He has detailed information about the glycemic index of foods and why high glycemic index foods promote aging. He also has chapters on various types of illness and tailors food and supplement intake for these groups of folks.

In Summary

Each of the books I have listed contains a wealth of information about each of these diets. These books detail shopping, food preparation, and cooking. If any of these approaches to food and eating appeal to you, I recommend you look for a book on it at your local library or book store. Always remember, when you try these diets, there is no one diet that will work wonderfully for every person because all of us are biochemically unique individuals. Just because your sister-in-law or co-worker does well on a certain diet does not necessarily mean that you will do well on that diet. As you have listened to this tape, you have probably noticed some similarities. Almost all of these diets emphasize liberal use of vegetables and fruits. As I said on previous tapes in this series, if I could get my patients to eat more vegetables and fruits without the sugar and fat that a lot of us include with those foods, that would make me very happy.

Dr. Honeyman's Opinions

I have some of my own opinions regarding these diets. First, the Fit for Life Diet, I think this is excellent especially in its reliance on fruits and vegetables. One problem that people in colder climates may have with this is that 70% raw fruits and vegetables may not give people enough calories, carbohydrates, and fats to keep warm in cold weather. The Fit for Life Diet is not appropriate for folks with diabetes or hypoglycemia. The macrobiotic diet is an excellent diet that has withstood the test of time in terms of improving people's health. If you try a macrobiotic diet and do not feel well on it, I would recommend that you seek out a health care practitioner who is skilled in tailoring macrobiotic diets to people's specific health needs.

I do not recommend the candida diet as a long-term diet because it is very high in protein. Diets high in protein put an undue burden on the kidneys. Additionally, if a few weeks of the candida diet does not take care of the problem for folks with candida, you need to seek out a health care practitioner who will apply other approaches to the candida.

Diets like the McDougall Plan and the Ornish Diet are very low in fat and low in animal protein and have also stood the test of time in reducing heart disease and cholesterol in many patients. For many folks, unless you are very careful to eat fresh whole grains and *no* refined grain products or flours, these diets risk deficiencies of essential fatty acids.

Many health care practitioners have reservations about the Zone Diet because of the relatively high percentage of protein compared to carbohydrate in the diet. Again, this is a definite concern for people with kidney problems as well as for elderly folks. Proportions of foods recommended in the blood type diets in terms of protein, fat, and carbohydrates are consistent with other healthy diets, and I also encourage my patients to experiment with the diet that is recommended for their blood type.

Dr. Honeyman's Favorite Diet

I recommend the phytonutrient detoxification diet most often for my patients. Many of the people coming to my practice don't feel well, in fact they often feel quite rotten, but don't have any disease the medical profession can diagnose. After a careful history and exam I often discover that they have impaired liver detoxification function with a high burden of toxic metals or other toxic compounds in their bodies. The phytonutrient diet along with a good quality multi-vitamin multi-mineral can go a long way to help these folks feel almost normal again.

Dr. Honeyman's "Bottom Line" in Eating

I'd like to state some basics for eating healthily. These are my "bottom line" if you will. First, I recommend we avoid toxins that we tend to take for granted in our food and water supply. Clean water is very important. Chlorine and certain micro organisms that survive chlorine are a definite problem in municipal water systems. Water filtered through a solid carbon block is probably the easiest way of obtaining pure water for most folks. Other waters free of contaminants are distilled water and reverse osmosis water. Municipalities should test water for volatile organic chemicals, known as VOC's. VOC's are often residues of manufacturing, the chemical industry, and farm chemicals. Municipal water systems often don't, but should, test for toxic minerals and should report it to the community on a regular basis. If you are using well water, you should know what is in it. Look for an analytical laboratory in your area that can test your well water for bacteria, arsenic, nitrites, and nitrates as a minimum. Well water can and should be tested for VOC's and toxic minerals.

Food crops grown with chemical fertilizers tend to be devoid of nutrients. If sewage sludge is used to fertilize them, this is high in heavy metals like cadmium which are absorbed into the plant and then eaten by us. Genetically engineered crops are much higher in herbicide residues than crops whose genetic material has not been tampered with, because they are genetically engineered to handle applications of twice as much herbicide. Another pitfall of genetically engineered crops is that often genes of other plants are added to genetically engineered plants. For example, if a wheat gene is added to a soy crop, a person not allergic to soy but who is allergic to wheat would probably have an allergic reaction to soy containing the wheat gene.

Look for grains, beans, fruits, and vegetables that have been organically grown. Refined grains and refined sugar strip our bodies of nutrients while being metabolized. On Tape 3, I gave you a list of food crops that are particularly high in pesticide and herbicide toxic residues. Again, that list is apples, apricots, grapes, peaches, cherries, spinach, bell peppers, celery, strawberries, wheat, green beans, and peanuts.

Dairy, beef animals, and poultry are routinely given antibiotics and hormones. The residues of these drugs are problematic for human beings eating them. Additionally, animals fed antibiotics have antibiotic resistant E-coli. These resistant strains of E-coli can be passed on to human beings causing virulent infections. In very young or very old folks these strains of E-coli can actually cause death.

Chemicals added to foods are problematic for our bodies. If a compound does not occur naturally, we should probably not be eating it. Preservatives are added to foods to prevent digestion of the foods by micro organisms. These preservatives prevent us from properly digesting the foods. Nutrasweet can cause inflammation of the membranes around the brain, headaches, or abnormal compounds in the brain. Aside from either Nutrasweet or sugar, soft drinks are high in phosphorus which disrupts calcium metabolism and contributes to osteoporosis.

Regarding fats and oils, remember, consume *no cotton seed oil*. Cotton is a non-food crop and much more toxic chemicals are used on cotton than are allowed on food crops. These toxins will concentrate in cotton seeds. Next, please do not eat hydrogenated oils. These are common ingredients in packaged foods; watch out for them! Olestra is not a naturally occurring molecule. It depletes the fat soluble vitamins: A, D, E, and K. Olestra has not been around long enough for us to determine what long-term effects it may have, but it certainly has been shown to cause diarrhea. Remember, diarrhea will disrupt the colonic flora leading to other serious health effects.

Toxic chemicals enter our food from the packaging. As much as possible buy fresh fruits, vegetables, and grains that do not need packaging. Especially problematic examples are aluminum in contact with tomato or any acidic food. Do not buy juices, etc., in aluminum cans. Plastic packaging in contact with food is also a problem. Especially toxic forms of plastic are the microwavable packaged foods you buy in the plastic package and stick right in the microwave. These have been shown to create toxic compounds in the food where the plastic contacts the food during the microwaving.

Foods to Include

After giving you so many "don'ts," let's talk about some of the do's. Good quality fats are very important for the health of the brain, spinal cord, and liver. These include olive oil, organic butter, flaxseed, and wild fish, especially salmon. Fresh foods are much better than processed foods or packaged foods. Eat from the perimeter of the supermarket. Eat fresh or frozen vegetables and fruits rather than canned vegetables and fruits. With fruits, drying is acceptable. Eat in restaurants that serve organic produce. As much as possible, buy foods that are organically grown. Consuming organically grown grains, beans, fruits, and vegetables is the easiest way to eliminate pesticide and herbicide residues from our diets.

If you eat meats, look for meats that are hormone and antibiotic free as a minimum. Better yet, look for grass-fed or free-range beef and poultry. Make sure you get your eggs from free-range chickens, and get organic dairy products. Dairy products from cows that have been fed only organic food and are hormone and antibiotic free are fairly easily available.

When buying packaged foods, please look for the least toxic packaging as well as ingredients. Tin cans are better than aluminum. Glass or cardboard containers are better than plastic. Acidic foods react the most with metals, especially aluminum. If you are buying citrus juice or tomato juice or sauce get them in glass. Don't buy ketchup in plastic, or tomato juice in aluminum cans. If you order juice in a restaurant ask if it comes in aluminum - you will find it usually does!

When I talk about food and diet with my patients, if they will at least follow this list I am happy:

- eat one to two cups vegetables every day
- eat the equivalent of three pieces of fruit every day
- substitute rice for at least one wheat serving daily
- eliminate or drastically cut back on sodapop
- eliminate Nutrasweet
- drastically cut back on sugar, raw and refined
- reduce meat to no more than 8 oz per day, try adding tofu occasionally
- deep fried foods or fast foods on very rare occasions, like 4 times a year
- no hydrogenated oils or cottonseed oil
- no food cooked or stored in aluminum

So, try this list and see if it makes you happy too!

Thanks for listening to Free to Be Well©! I hope you are enjoying this series, and most of all I hope you have learned lots of useful information.

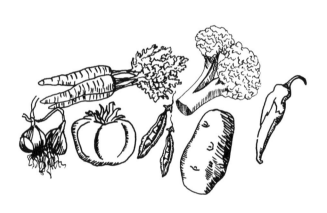

Chapter 5
Glad Glands

Hello, and welcome to the fifth tape in our series Free to Be Well[©]. On this tape I am going to talk about the endocrine system, conditions specific to women and osteoporosis, and for men I will be talking about benign prostatic hypertrophy. The endocrine system is a collection of glands that make hormones. The main gland in the endocrine system is the pituitary located just underneath the center of the brain. It makes many hormones that regulate the rate of activity of each of our other glands. The thyroid gland is located in the front of the throat, the adrenal glands sit like little caps on top of the kidneys, the pancreas which is behind the stomach has special cells that make hormones, the ovaries sit roughly on either side of the bladder, and the testes, or testicles sit below the bladder outside the body.

Hormones are either protein or cholesterol-based ring structures that are made by one tissue and travel through the body and affect another target tissue. There is a complex interplay of constant feedback among the hormones; many of them increase or decrease secretion of other hormones. In addition to these glands that I have listed above, we also make hormones in the liver, stomach, and intestinal lining.

Science is discovering that many cells in our body make hormones. In fact, many of the same hormones that are made by our endocrine glands are also made by the central nervous system, brain, spinal cord, and other tissues in the body. Endocrinologists, folks who study glands, call these substances hormones. Neuroscientists, folks who study the brain and spinal cord, call the same exact chemicals neuropeptides instead of hormones. Again, a hormone is a chemical made by one tissue or organ which stimulates a receptor in another tissue or organ resulting in cellular changes in the target tissue.

Endocrine Glands

Endocrine glands make hormones which travel in the blood stream and affect other organs. Each gland and its hormone has a different purpose. The pituitary gland makes many of the hormones that tell the other glands to make their respective hormones. Thyroid hormone is responsible for our metabolic rate. That is, how fast our cells burn energy. The adrenal glands make adrenalin, the fight or flight hormone, corticosteroids, DHEA, and a few other hormones. The endocrine cells of the pancreas make insulin which keeps our blood sugar from getting too high. They also make glucagon which helps keep our blood sugar high enough between meals. The ovaries make estrogen, progesterone, and testosterone - yes, women have testosterone, and men have estrogen, too! The testicles make testosterone and estrogen. To make their hormones, endocrine glands depend on cholesterol and proteins supplied by the liver. Almost invariably, if the liver is happy and healthy, the endocrine glands will be happy too.

Thyroid Gland

I would like to talk about each of the major glands and what their hormones do in the body. The thyroid gland is the keeper of our energy! The thyroid gland is actually the largest endocrine gland and is responsible for our metabolic rate. In other words, the thyroid gland controls how fast our cells burn energy and how fast each of our respective cells does its own job. The thyroid gland can effectively put all of our body's cells on fast forward or slow them down and put them in slow motion depending on how much hormone it puts out into the blood stream. The gland is located in the neck below the voice box and on both sides of the windpipe. Its hormone, thyroxine, circulates in our bloodstream and tells all our cells how fast to work and how fast to do their jobs.

Getting thyroxine to our cells depends on how much thyroxine the thyroid gland makes and on how much thyroglobulin the liver makes. Thyroglobulin is a large protein whose job is transporting thyroxine in the blood stream. This protein is made specifically for this purpose. In order for our livers to make thyroglobulin, we need to have tyrosine and glutamine which are two amino acids. Normal thyroid function can be encouraged by the supplementation of tyrosine and glutamine combined as tyromine. If our liver cannot make enough thyroglobulin, then the thyroxine (thyroid hormone) does not get transported in our blood stream to the cells and the cells do not get enough of the thyroxine to keep doing their job at an adequate speed. In other words, without enough thyroglobulin, our cells will slow down in the same way that they do if we do not have enough thyroxine. Iodine is part of thyroxine, the thyroid gland's hormone. The thyroid gland depends on iodine in the body in order to make enough thyroxine.

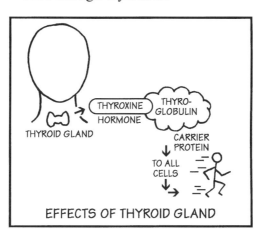

EFFECTS OF THYROID GLAND

Food allergies or delayed sensitivities will frequently affect thyroid function via the immune system. They can cause the thyroid to make consistently less thyroxine to fluctuate between inadequate output of thyroxine and excess output, usually over a span of several weeks. So a patient will have several weeks of decreased thyroid function and then several weeks of increased thyroid function when they have lots and lots of energy. The thyroid gland is very sensitive to the state of the immune system. If one is hyper allergic because of a poor diet, chronic inflammation, or airborne allergies, this can often affect thyroid function. I have seen patients with either low thyroid function or fluctuating thyroid function regain normal function once they have eliminated the foods they are sensitive to from their diet. In my experience anything that causes the immune system to get irritated and over reactive can also affect thyroid function. There are also a variety of medications that affect thyroid function. I will give you a list so that if you are taking any of these medications, you can be aware of this specific side effect. Asthma medications, corticosteroids (drugs like Prednisone), oral contraceptives, and hormone replacement all affect the thyroid gland. I would like to note here that, as I have done on previous tapes, I will talk about how to keep the endocrine system healthy at the end of this tape.

Pancreas

Next let's talk about the pancreas. Remember, on Tape Two, I talked about enzymes the pancreas makes for digestion. The pancreas has two different types of cells, cells that make digestive enzymes that are excreted into the intestinal tract and cells that make hormones that are secreted into the blood stream. It is the cells that make the hormones that I will be discussing on this tape.

The two main hormones of the pancreas are insulin and glucagon. Insulin, as most of us know, is the hormone responsible for moving sugar from the blood stream into our cells. Insulin release from pancreatic cells is dependent on calcium, so calcium levels in the blood can affect insulin levels. When we eat food our blood sugar rises as the carbohydrates from the food enter the blood stream. In response, the pancreas secretes insulin, and insulin levels in the blood stream rise within 10 minutes of eating. With the rise in insulin, sugar in the blood moves into our cells for energy use, and blood sugar levels drop. Blood sugar should return to normal two hours after meals. So, insulin is finished with its job within two hours of each meal we eat.

We can keep insulin high by eating every two hours, especially if we eat sweets or drink sweet beverages like juice or soda. With the continuous presence of sugars in the blood stream, from starches and sweets we eat, the pancreas gets desensitized and eventually stops secreting enough insulin.

We need more than just insulin to get sugar from the blood stream into our cells. The activity of insulin to move sugar into cells depends on insulin receptors in the cell membrane. Insulin receptors transport glucose across the cell membrane from the blood stream to the inside of the cell. Chromium will help increase the number of these insulin receptors. If my insulin runs too high or too low or I have too few insulin receptors I will have abnormal blood sugar levels. Low blood sugar is much more uncomfortable and dangerous for the brain than

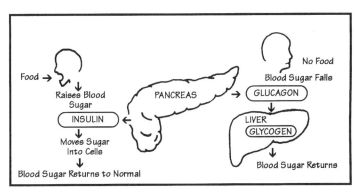

THE ENDOCRINE PANCREAS

high blood sugar.

Insulin's job is to facilitate storage of nutrients inside cells. It causes liver and muscle cells to make more glycogen which is the way those cells store sugar for energy use later. Insulin will increase triglycerides, the levels of fat in the blood. Insulin also increases cholesterol and VLDL cholesterol, the very bad cholesterol. Elevated insulin inhibits the secretion of glucagon, which we will talk about shortly. In addition to increasing the level of triglycerides and cholesterol in the blood, insulin

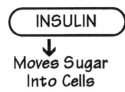

also promotes manufacture and storage of triglycerides in fat cells and discourages fat cells from releasing fat for energy use. This pattern of elevated insulin, high cholesterol, and triglycerides is called Syndrome X, which we will talk about shortly.

The other major hormone made by the pancreas is glucagon. In many ways insulin and glucagon are mirror images of each other. The main job of glucagon is to make energy available to tissues between meals. Remember that insulin will rise after we eat, mobilize sugar in our blood into the cells and then, once blood sugar drops, insulin levels also drop. Glucagon, on the other hand, has the job of keeping blood sugar from dropping too low before the next meal. Glucagon stimulates the body to break down glycogen stored in the liver for energy. It also gets the liver to make sugar from protein and ketone bodies for energy from fat. Glucagon promotes the use of fat present in the liver for energy. The release of insulin is stimulated by eating refined starches and sugars, conversely the release of glucagon will be stimulated by eating protein. We don't release insulin and glucagon at the same time. If blood

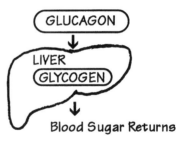

sugar and triglycerides are elevated, release of glucagon is inhibited.

Insulin affects the liver, muscles, and fat tissues by getting them to store more glycogen and triglycerides (or fat) for energy use later. Glucagon really only affects the liver, but does not change the metabolism of fat cells. Glucagon gets the liver to use the fat stored in the liver for energy, but it does not mobilize fat from fat cells.

A third hormone released by the pancreas with insulin is somatostatin. This hormone slows digestion in the stomach and decreases pancreatic enzyme secretion. Somatostatin also slows down nutrient absorption from the small intestine into the blood stream. Because insulin and somatostatin are secreted into the blood stream together, release of insulin will also slow digestion and absorption of nutrients.

In order to keep the endocrine cells of the pancreas healthy over the long term it is vital to eat properly. The way to use diet to best keep these hormones in line and the pancreas happy is to drastically limit or eliminate refined sweets like candies, pastries, pies, cakes, cookies, ice cream, soda pop, etc. Refined carbohydrates like white flour products and alcohol must also be limited or eliminated from our diets. These foods are the most destructive foods in terms of the hormone balance of insulin, somatostatin, and glucagon in the blood stream.

Syndrome X

I would like to talk briefly about Syndrome X. Researchers have noticed there is a relationship of various factors in some individuals: high insulin in the blood stream, high blood sugar, high fats in the blood (cholesterol and triglycerides), and high blood pressure. These conditions in combination increase the likelihood of heart disease and stroke much more than any of these conditions alone will. People who have this combination of high blood sugar, high cholesterol and triglycerides, high insulin, and high blood pressure are much more likely to develop non-insulin-dependent diabetes. This is commonly known as adult onset diabetes. Folks predisposed to adult onset diabetes usually have insulin resistance. Insulin resistance means the pancreas is responding to the high blood sugar by secreting more insulin but the sugar is not moving from the blood stream into the cells. Many researchers believe the resistance of cells to insulin's efforts to move sugar into cells is the cause of Syndrome X.

Let's look at what factors cause insulin resistance because it can result in high cholesterol, high triglycerides, and high blood pressure as well as high blood sugar. Prolonged high blood sugar causes insulin resistance. Folks who eat lots of sweets, white flour products, and alcohol will have prolonged high blood sugar which will predispose them to diabetes. Diseases of the liver or adrenal glands cause insulin resistance. Drugs like Prednisone, corticosteroids, oral contraceptives, progesterone, growth hormone, and thyroxine (or synthroid) can each cause insulin resistance and predispose people to adult onset diabetes.

A sedentary lifestyle or lack of exercise contributes to insulin resistance. As you can see, prevention of insulin resistance and diabetes primarily involves factors within our control. Diabetes is a devastating disease that is increasingly common in North America.

Blood Sugar Control

Most of us know that diabetes is a disease involving the loss of blood sugar control with consistent episodes of high blood sugar. Hypoglycemia is a condition with low blood sugar. Hypoglycemics often get light headed or irritable when their blood sugar is low. This is because our brain cells use sugar as their main energy source. What many of us don't know is that tight blood sugar control in diabetes causes episodes of low blood sugar that are dangerous for the brain. These episodes deprive brain cells of nutrition which can cause some brain cells to die. I am not talking about the extremely low blood sugar in a diabetic person who takes insulin and fails to eat causing insulin shock, which can be fatal. I'm referring to the mildly low blood sugar that can make a diabetic woozy or foggy headed. Insulin shock is also bad for the brain, it just isn't as common as low blood sugar.

I will talk at the end of this tape about nutritional supplements that help prevent the development of hormonal problems with the pancreas.

Adrenal Glands

Adrenal glands are little caps sitting on top of our kidneys and primarily manage fluids, blood pressure, and stress! The adrenal glands have an outer cortex which makes the hormones cortisol, the androgens (male type hormones), and aldosterone. The inner medulla, the center portion of the adrenal glands, makes epinephrine, norepinephrine, and dopamine. Epinephrine and norepinephrine are also known as adrenalin. When people talk about an adrenalin rush they really mean the release of epinephrine or norepinephrine.

Medulla- Dopamine, Epinephrine, Norepinephrine

I'll talk first about the hormones of the adrenal medulla, dopamine, epinephrine, and norepinephrine. Two of these hormones, dopamine and norepinephrine, are made in the brain and spinal cord and by the sympathetic nervous system as well as by the adrenal medulla. The sympathetic nervous system governs our "fight or flight" response. This is an example of the similarities between endocrine and brain function. Manufacture of dopamine, norepinephrine and epinephrine starts from an amino acid, tyrosine. These hormones are made and stored principally in the adrenal glands. They are released as needed. They are part of our normal "fight or flight" response and will be released in a burst if we are put in danger or frightened by something. Proper storage of these hormones requires adequate calcium and magnesium.

These three hormones dopamine, norepinephrine, and epinephrine are also known as catecholamines and are released secondary to a variety of stressful experiences: things like surgery, heart pain, heart attack, hemorrhage, hypoglycemia, lack of oxygen, etc. Most of our cells have receptors for epinephrine and norepinephrine. When these receptors get stimulated by the presence of these hormones, the effects vary depending on which hormone stimulated which receptor of the cell. These hormones of 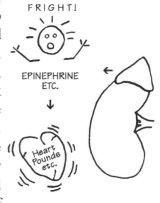 the adrenal medulla have a variety of effects on our bodies. Most noticeable to us, they increase the force and rate of the heart beat. This is what causes the feeling of your heart pounding in your chest. These hormones dilate or constrict blood vessels depending on which blood vessels they are affecting. They open bronchial airways, and increase the breakdown of fats and glycogen for energy. In the gut, epinephrine and norepinephrine can slow or stop digestion by slowing the contractions that move food through the intestines and increasing gut sphincter tone. This is what causes us to feel our bellies tighten during that adrenalin rush. Depending on whether epinephrine or norepinephrine is secreted it will either decrease insulin and glucagon or increase insulin and glucagon. Epinephrine and norepinephrine literally make us sweat. They increase our need for oxygen and make our bodies heat up. Epinephrine and norepinephrine, or adrenalin, also influence whether or not the kidney keeps or dumps sodium, water, calcium, potassium, and phosphate.

Stimulant substances like over-the-counter drugs for weight loss or herbal products for weight loss with the herb Ephedra or Ma Huang cause constant stimulation of the sympathetic nervous system. They simulate the effect of constant adrenalin secretion. This is extremely hard on people's hearts, and the use of these products is not good for long-term health.

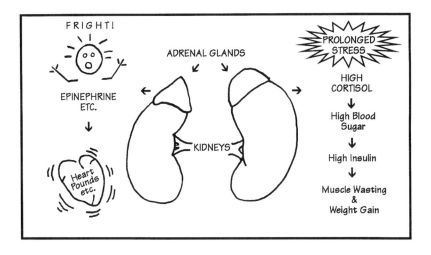

Adrenal Cortex

Moving on to the adrenal cortex, these hormones are cortisol, the androgens ("male" hormones), and aldosterone. The manufacture of each of these hormones begins with cholesterol. To adequately manufacture these hormones, the adrenal glands depend upon adequate cholesterol in the blood stream. Cholesterol is the foundation from which most of our body's hormones are made. Progesterone, which is also made from cholesterol, is an intermediate step when the adrenal cortex makes cortisol and aldosterone.

Cortisol

Cortisol is the most commonly known adrenal cortical hormone. It helps maintain blood sugar when we are fasting. Many people use corticosteroid medications which are synthetic versions of cortisol. Prednisone, which is commonly used for asthma, is one of these medications. Natural cortisol has several functions in the body. It increases the body's production of sugar from protein and it also increases the storage

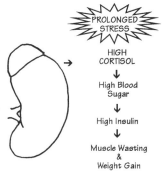

PROLONGED STRESS

HIGH CORTISOL
↓
High Blood Sugar
↓
High Insulin
↓
Muscle Wasting & Weight Gain

of glycogen in the liver and muscle cells. Cortisol increases the production in the liver of sugar and protein, and in muscle cells cortisol decreases the uptake of sugar and protein into the cell and increases the release of amino acids (protein building blocks) into the blood stream from muscle tissue. Because cortisol inhibits muscles from getting protein and sugar from the blood and makes muscles release their protein into the blood stream it causes muscle breakdown over time. In fat tissue cortisol stimulates the breakdown of fat for energy, but it also causes fat to accumulate around the face, trunk, neck, and belly. People who have been on Prednisone for a long time or have a natural excess secretion of cortisol will have a round face and large trunk with thin arms and legs. The reason for this unusual deposition of fat is not known.

Lack of cortisol secretion by the adrenal glands will cause low blood sugar, fatigue, depression, and irritability. Irritability happens because the brain depends on sugar in the blood for energy. When it doesn't have enough blood sugar, people get irritable. An excess of cortisol can cause high blood sugar, high insulin, muscle wasting, weight gain with the unusual fat distribution that I talked about, thinning of skin, and osteoporosis. Cortisol hormones also decrease the absorption of calcium and increase calcium excretion in the urine. This is how they cause osteoporosis. These hormones also raise blood pressure and interfere with immune system function. They cause impaired memory and concentration and may cause cataracts. All of these symptoms that I just listed are caused either by a natural excess of cortisol (which is rare) or by prescription drugs like Prednisone.

Aldosterone

The next adrenal cortical hormone that I would like to talk about is aldosterone. Aldosterone maintains sodium and potassium levels and fluid in the spaces between our cells. We have fluid in our blood stream and we have fluid in the capillary beds that bathe all our cells. Nutrients have to go from the capillaries, the tiniest blood vessels, into the space between the cells where the fluid is. The regulation of sodium and potassium in these fluid spaces is very important. Aldosterone tells the kidneys to keep sodium in the body. When the kidneys are making urine, there are complex decisions they make constantly about keeping or dumping sodium, potassium, calcium, phosphorus, or magnesium. Aldosterone causes us to keep sodium and fluid in our body and excrete potassium into the urine. Aldosterone increases blood pressure. We can increase aldosterone levels with licorice candy or herb which will, over time, raise blood pressure. A diet consistently high in salt will promote the loss of potassium in the urine and, conversely, a diet low in salt will tend to save potassium. The abuse of laxatives or diuretics can cause an increase in aldosterone which will cause an increase in fluid retention. Dehydration will elevate aldosterone to help the body conserve fluids.

To maintain normal aldosterone levels, don't eat a diet high in salt. Salt in moderation is fine. Don't use licorice on a regular basis, either medicinally or as a food or candy. Don't use diuretics or laxatives on a regular basis. Again, this advice is for people who do not have a disease where they need to be taking prescription medications like diuretics.

Androgens

The last type of adrenal cortical hormones are the adrenal androgens. These are considered male hormones. However, women and men both normally have androgens, estrogen, and progesterone. Everyone has both "female" and "male" hormones. In fact, men without progesterone or estrogen develop severe osteoporosis.

The list of adrenal androgens includes DHEA, DHEA sulfate, androstenedione, and testosterone. The popular supplement, DHEA, is an adrenal androgen. All of these are made from pregnenolone and progesterone which are made from cholesterol. Cholesterol is the starting substance for each of these adrenal androgens as well as for aldosterone and cortisol we just talked about. The function of these androgen hormones is unknown. They serve as precursors to testosterone in both men and women. In men the effect of adrenal androgens is minimal because men make much more testosterone in their testicles. In women the adrenal androgens normally account for about 50% of circulating testosterone and the ovaries make the other 50%. As I said, the function of these hormones is unknown. Women with excess adrenal androgen production will have signs of masculinization like acne and facial hair. These physical signs can be a side effect of DHEA supplementation in women. There are varying recommendations for DHEA supplementation. I generally do not like to see women or men take more than 10 mg per day of DHEA until they know whether they tolerate it. Certainly if a woman is using DHEA and is noticing facial hair growth, she is taking too much. I will talk at the end of this tape about nutritional support for proper adrenal gland function.

Female Hormones

Then next area I would like to discuss is female hormones, women's conditions, and osteoporosis. Female hormones are made primarily by women's ovaries. Our ovaries make estrogens, progesterone, androgens including testosterone, relaxin, and prostaglandins. The starting substance from which all these are synthesized is cholesterol, so again cholesterol is very important. Cholesterol is transformed into the hormone pregnenolone, then to progesterone, then to androstenedione and testosterone, and finally the androstenedione and testosterone are made into the estrogens. Women have circulating testosterone because it is an intermediary step in making estrogen.

Estrogens

Estrogens are responsible for the female sexual characteristics. They are responsible for the development of the uterus, vagina, breasts, and body fat distribution. All of the changes with a girl's puberty are caused and maintained by the presence of estrogens. Estrogens decrease bone resorption and they decrease bowel motility. I have patients who have been on synthetic hormone replacement therapy and develop trouble with spasms of their esophagus or swallowing trouble after starting estrogen. This is because estrogens decrease the motility or muscle contraction that happens in the esophagus, stomach, and intestines. Estrogens enhance clotting of blood, so high estrogen levels can cause stroke. Estrogens increase the good cholesterol, HDL cholesterol. Estrogens can cause the swelling and sodium and water retention which many of us are familiar with.

Progesterone

Progesterone is the other main female hormone. Progesterone causes the glandular development of the breasts, cyclical thickening of the lining of the uterus during the menstrual period, increases body temperature, increases bone mineral density, increases insulin, and decreases sodium retention. For women who tend toward bloating premenstrually, they often have higher estrogen levels in relation to progesterone.

Hormone Levels Through the Menstrual Cycle

Let's talk about the normal menstrual cycle, because estrogen and progesterone levels normally fluctuate throughout the month. Technically the menstrual cycle starts with the first day of the menstrual period. During menstruation both progesterone and estrogen are low. Those hormones are both at the lowest levels throughout the cycle during menstruation. Ovulation is the release of the ripened egg or ovum from the ovary, and it happens fourteen days before the next menstrual period. Before ovulation, estrogen gradually rises until it normally peaks about one or two days prior to ovulation. Then it drops slowly until it bottoms out during the next menstrual period. After ovulation progesterone begins to rise for about one week and then falls for another week. Then, progesterone bottoms out during menstruation. Remember progesterone causes the thickening of the lining of the uterus. When progesterone drops off, menstruation starts. Menstruation is the shedding of the lining of the uterus.

An approximation of what happens with hormones during the menstrual period is that estrogen peaks between menstruation and ovulation and progesterone peaks between ovulation and menstruation. To say it another way, estrogen should be high during the first half of the menstrual cycle prior to ovulation and progesterone should be higher during the second half of the cycle after ovulation. This is our introduction to the next topic: PMS or premenstrual syndrome.

PMS

Premenstrual syndrome is any symptoms that happen regularly between ovulation and menstruation and stop when menstruation starts. There are a galaxy of symptoms that can happen. Remember that estrogen and progesterone drop drastically during menstruation, so when these hormone levels both fall, the symptoms of PMS disappear. Symptoms of PMS may be emotional, physical, or both. Some women have primarily emotional symptoms. These can be irritability, anxiety, or depression. Other women have mainly physical symptoms. Physical symptoms are those caused by fluid retention. This includes weight gain, bloating, breast tenderness, and headaches. Whether the symptoms are emotional or physical, they can vary greatly in intensity from one woman to the next. I have seen patients with such bad PMS that for one or two days a month they are almost suicidal or they have fits of uncontrollable rage. When we did blood tests on one of my patients with these symptoms, we found she was slightly hypothyroid and deficient in essential fatty acids. With the appropriate nutritional supplements she was fine in time for her next menstrual period. This particular woman's PMS had worsened after both of her pregnancies. Incidentally, moms become more deficient in essential fatty acids with each child that they bear. Her PMS was primarily a deficiency of essential fatty acids.

The cause of PMS is thought to be due to an imbalance between estrogen and progesterone levels before menstruation. After ovulation there is an imbalance in the amount of estrogen and progesterone. Some women who have PMS have too much estrogen (remember estrogen is supposed to be dropping after ovulation), and other women with PMS have progesterone levels that are too high in relation to the amount of circulating estrogens. One approach to prevention of PMS is the use of herbs that are either estrogenic or progesterogenic. These are herbs that provide estrogen precursors for the body to make estrogens with and/or herbs that provide progesterone precursors for the body to make progesterones with. The principle progesterone promoting herb is Wild Yam. Some of the common herbs used to promote estrogen are the Chinese herb Dong quai, Black Cohosh, and Licorice. Soy proteins, especially the proteins available in tofu and tempeh, are rich with hormone precursors for both estrogen and progesterone, so they serve to balance both hormones. We will talk a bit more about this at the end of this tape.

Dysmenorrhea

Dysmenorrhea is a Latin word. Menorrhea means menstruation and dys means bad. The word dysmenorrhea means difficult menstruation, and this includes any symptoms that are intense enough to interfere with a woman's normal activities. The usual symptoms of dysmenorrhea that many of us are familiar with are intense cramping, heavy bleeding, and low-back pain. Remember progesterone and estrogen are low during menstruation. The symptoms of dysmenorrhea are usually caused by prostaglandins. Prostaglandins are hormones made by white blood cells and many other cells of the body. Prostaglandins are responsible for inflammation. Essential fatty acid deficiency will increase inflammatory prostaglandins in the body.

Menopause

Next I would like to briefly discuss menopause. Menopause is also known as the climacteric and it refers to the years of a woman's life during which her menstrual periods and the ripening of ova every month cease. During this time most women will have gradual changes in menstrual cycles with a decrease in the amount and length of flow and irregularity of cycles. Some women will experience more frequent cycles with heavier bleeding, although this is less common. A minority of women will just abruptly stop menstruating. Most of my patients do not miss their menstrual periods. It is the other symptoms that go along with the climacteric that bother women. The principle thing that bothers most women is hot flashes, or as some of my patients call them, power surges. These can be most troublesome when they occur at night. Because of the night sweats and discomfort that accompanies them, many women develop insomnia. They are woken up sometimes as often as every hour with these hot flashes.

Other problems that bother women during menopause include headaches, depression, mental function problems, cognitive (or thinking) problems, and also problems related to thinning of the mucosal lining of the vagina and urethra. Because of the drop in estrogen and progesterone, women are more likely to develop osteoporosis and heart disease after menopause than prior to menopause. These conditions are asymptomatic until later, but prevention is always the better part of dealing with these. I will talk about nutritional prevention of menopausal symptoms at the end of this tape. However, remember that the information I gave in Tape One of this series about preventing heart and blood vessel disease is particularly applicable for women as we traverse the climacteric.

Osteoporosis

Osteoporosis occurs as bones become less dense or even brittle. There is a gradual decline in bone density that occurs as we age for both men and women. In women the greatest accelerated loss of bone density happens with the drop in estrogen and progesterone during the climacteric or menopause. The loss of bone with osteoporosis is a very long, slow process. In women, it starts in the mid to late 30's and there is a gradual loss of bone that accelerates with menopause. Often we are unaware that we have osteoporosis until we actually break a bone. We have all heard of elderly women who fall and fracture their hip. With advanced osteoporosis in an elderly person, these fractures may never heal which creates a disability for the rest of that individual's life. The best treatment for osteoporosis is prevention!

Men

Men have the hormones testosterone, dihydrotestosterone, and estradiol. These are all made from cholesterol. In men, 90% of testosterone is made in the testicles and 80% of the dihydrotestosterone and estradiol come from conversion in other organs of the hormones made by the adrenal glands and testicles. The male glands or testes make sperm. The ducts from each of the testicles meet at the prostate gland which is located between the bones that we sit on, roughly where women have a vagina is where men have a prostate gland. The prostate gland adds fluid to the semen. An interesting fact to know is that semen contains Vitamin C, flavonoid type compounds that are parts of fruits and vegetables, choline which is a B vitamin, the mineral zinc, and phospholipids. Testicles make sperm and the prostate adds more fluid to the semen when it comes from the testicles. This brings us to a discussion of benign prostatic hypertrophy (BPH).

What is BPH?

Benign prostatic hypertrophy is the hardening and enlargement in the prostate gland that occurs almost universally in Western countries (North America and Europe) when men get to be over 55 or 60 years of age. This benign prostatic hypertrophy makes it more difficult for men to start their urinary stream and it also makes it more difficult for them to fully empty their bladder. Many men have to get up more than once during the night to urinate because their bladder remains partially filled. In Benign Prostatic Hypertrophy the prostate gland continues to grow and harden. Basically what the prostate gland does is squish the urethra which is why men have trouble with urination. This enlargement and hardening of the prostate gland is usually secondary to excess dihydrotestosterone. The dihydrotestosterone is generally a product of the peripheral conversion by the adrenal glands and other tissues in the body rather than a direct product of the testicles. As men age, they make proportionally more of this dihydrotestosterone and this stimulates the cells of the prostate gland.

The increased levels of this secondary testosterone [dihydro-testosterone] are responsible not only for benign prostatic hypertrophy, but also for male pattern balding. Improving hormone metabolism generally as well as improving these hormone pathways may also help prevent male pattern balding.

Nutritional Prevention

At this point I would like to move on to nutritional prevention of some of the endocrine diseases we have talked about on this tape. First of all I would like to talk generally about the endocrine system and things that all of our endocrine glands need. As we have seen, cholesterol forms the foundation building block for many of these endocrine hormones. In order for the liver to have normal cholesterol metabolism, it has to be healthy and happy. That goes back to all the things we have talked about on previous tapes which are: good quality multi-vitamin multi-mineral, make sure the liver has enough B vitamins, that it has enough antioxidants like beta-carotene, vitamin C, vitamin E, and also that the liver has enough minerals, calcium, magnesium, selenium, iron, chromium, etc.

Another point about liver health and endocrine problems is that alcoholism and liver disease will interfere with the normal function of our endocrine glands and either one of these two, alcoholism or liver disease, can cause feminization in men. In other words, liver disease or alcoholism will interfere enough with normal hormone metabolism that men will make more estrogen and less testosterone.

The next thing to enhance normal metabolism in the liver and endocrine system is the fats that we eat. The first consideration about fats is to eliminate bad fats from the diet. I have talked about those on previous tapes. Please don't eat hydrogenated fats, polyunsaturated vegetable oils, things like corn oil, soy oil, those generic see-through, clear vegetable oils in the supermarket. Any oil you can keep at room temperature and it never goes rancid is not healthy for the liver. So how do we get good fat in our diet? Good fat is extremely important for normal liver metabolism, normal cell membranes, and also for normal endocrine metabolism. All of us need essential fatty acids and we can get those from good quality oils, from nuts and seeds, or from fresh fish. The fins and scales type fish that I have mentioned on previous tapes are rich in essential fatty acids. I usually put my patients with really bad PMS on a combination of flax and borage oil in capsules or black currant seed oil. Anywhere from 3-4 capsules a day up to as many as 15 capsules a day may be needed to help prevent symptoms of endocrine problems if people are deficient in essential fatty acids. One way you can tell whether your body has enough omega 3's (which are present in flax oil) is if you have dry skin. If we have enough omega 3's in our diet, our skin should be soft, smooth, and velvety.

Another nutritional support for the endocrine system is soy isoflavones that I have mentioned previously on this tape. You can get soy isoflavones either in pill form or they are available in tofu and tempeh as foods. Soy isoflavones provide precursors to endocrine hormones including estrogen, progesterone, and testosterone. The body will chose to use these precursors wherever it needs the hormone. In other words, if a woman has too much estrogen, the soy isoflavones will actually get attached to estrogen receptors on cell sites and calm them down. It will block the stimulation by excess estrogen. On the other hand, if a woman does not have enough estrogen, the soy isoflavones attach to the cell receptors and stimulate them because the cell receptors for estrogen have not been stimulated by anything else. Soy does the same thing that I just described about estrogen metabolism and estrogen receptors with testosterone and testosterone receptors and progesterone and progesterone receptors. Incidently, in Asian countries where soy is a regular part of the diet from childhood on, problems like PMS, menopausal discomforts, and benign prostatic hypertrophy are virtually unknown. Having soy foods in the diet is an excellent long-term prevention for these problems.

Which brings me to the fourth vital aspect of keeping the endocrine system happy. Remember the information from Tape Two about gastrointestinal health and keeping the gut happy? There is a complex interplay between the cholesterol and hormones the liver dumps to the gall bladder (then to the intestine) and the bacteria in the large intestine. If we have good bugs lining the colon wall, then they will do their part in our hormone metabolism with these byproducts from the gall bladder. If we have an imbalance of the organisms in the colon, then we are likely to have PMS, dysmenorrhea, menopausal discomforts, BPH or a variety of other problems we discussed on Tape Two. The interesting thing about this is we can normalize the types of organisms present in the gut with regular use of freshly ground flax seed, and if the soy isoflavones don't work by themselves to prevent menopausal symptoms, the combination of soy isoflavones and flax seed almost always will work.

And lastly don't forget the importance of all those phytonutrients in vegetables and fruits! They are as vital to the health of the endocrine system as much as they are for the liver and gastrointestinal system! So remember to eat your veggies!

Thyroid

I would like to go back up to the beginning of our list of the endocrine glands and talk about each endocrine gland and nutritional things we can do help support their function. For thyroid function I talked about food allergies being a problem. Eliminating foods that cause general inflammation in the body will improve thyroid function as well. Iodine is very important to the thyroid gland for making thyroid hormone (thyroxine). An amino acid supplement called tyromine, which is a combination of the two amino acids, tyrosine and glutamine, is an important building block for the protein that carries thyroxine in the blood. We can augment normal thyroid function by supplementing with either full-spectrum amino acids or specifically tyromine.

Pancreas

Moving on to the pancreas and insulin and glucagon metabolism, diabetes is a devastating disease which is all too common in North America. Taking good care of our pancreas will prevent or diminish the severity of diabetes. The first line thing to do for the pancreas and keeping insulin metabolism normal is to eat a good quality diet. I talked at length on Tape Four about what the essence of a good quality diet is. Sugar and bad fats - poor quality fats in the diet are very hard on the pancreas. There are a lot of things we can do with nutritional supplements to help make the job of the pancreas easier in managing our blood sugar. The minerals chromium, vanadium, and lithium are all very important to blood sugar.

The easiest way I know to find out whether or not you are deficient in lithium is with a hair mineral analysis. Lithium is not generally included as part of a multi-vitamin multi-mineral. If you discover that you are deficient in lithium, you will need to get that as a separate supplement by itself. One or two mg per day of lithium is sufficient unless you are being supervised by a physician, and please don't use lithium unless you know you need it.

Chromium should be in a good quality multi-vitamin multi-mineral at about the level of 200 mcg per day. That is the minimum dose I like my healthy patients to be taking. It is thought that chromium increases the numbers of insulin receptors on the cell walls, thus making it easier for insulin to do its job in moving sugar into our cells from the blood stream. Vanadium improves cellular response to insulin and 200 mcg of vanadium should be in any good multi-vitamin multi-mineral. Vanadium is contraindicated for folks with bipolar disease as it displaces lithium.

Calcium is also important for the pancreas, I recommend folks get 300 to 800 mg per day of a good quality calcium. Zinc is vital for normal blood sugar handling, and its dose for adults is 15 to 20 mg per day. Be sure if you are using zinc that you also get at least 1 to 2 mg copper per day. These two minerals easily get out of balance. B-complex and lipoic acid are also very useful for normal sugar handling. I recommend 100 to 300 mg per day of lipoic acid and one or two capsules daily of a good B-complex.

Adrenals

The adrenal glands need several vitamins to keep them happy. These are vitamin A or beta-carotene, vitamin C, vitamin E, B6, B5 (aka pantothenic acid), and B12. Generally I recommend a good quality, good potency multivitamin mineral for my patients who can use adrenal support. This will often do the trick. Magnesium and calcium are also important for the adrenals. In some cases folks may find free form amino acids helpful as well.

Also remember occasional use of licorice is fine for the adrenals, but don't use it regularly. Please don't use ephedra or Ma Huang more than rarely either (i.e. once or twice a month).

Women's Hormones

For prevention of PMS, dysmenorrhea, and menopausal symptoms I recommend starting by ensuring you are not deficient in essential fatty acids. Most of us are. Remember we need fats to be healthy, and we need good quality fats. Don't forget that essential fatty acids are vital to the endocrine system. Most of us are deficient in the omega 3's and many of us are deficient in the omega 6's. Some sources of these are flax seeds for the omega 3's, sesame seeds, walnuts, and hemp seeds for a mixture of mainly omega 6's and some omega 3's. If you purchase these in oil form taste them to be sure they aren't rancid. The oil should taste like the seeds it came from. The dosage is 3 to 15 capsules daily or 1 to 3 tablespoons daily.

The proteins in soy are very beneficial for modulating estrogen and progesterone whether they are too high or too low. The dose of soy isoflavones is one third of a cake of tofu or tempeh daily or 500 to 1000 mg of supplemental soy isoflavones. Soy protein powders and soy milk do not have the isoflavones available to us.

Some estrogenic herbs are licorice (please don't use this daily), dong quai, and black cohosh (also available as the extract Remifemin). Some progesterogenic herbs are wild yam and sarsparilla, which should not be used long term on a regular basis. Last but not least Vitex agnus castus or chasteberry is a wonderful hormone balancer. It is thought to act on the pituitary and the ovaries and get them communicating with each other. Another balancing herb is false unicorn root.

The usual dosage on herbs is 3 cups of tea daily, 3 to 6 capsules daily, or sixty drops of liquid tincture daily.

Osteoporosis Prevention

Prevention of osteoporosis is much more than calcium, exercise, and prescription hormone replacement therapy.

First I'd like to discuss the lifestyle habits that cause bone loss by causing the kidneys to dump large amounts of calcium in the urine. With each 8 to 12 oz. cup of coffee whether it is caffeinated or decaf we lose 25 to 50 mg of calcium. The same is true for carbonated beverages, whether or not they contain caffeine. Other factors that promote bone loss are: alcohol, sugar and refined foods, cigarette smoking, and excessive sodium in the diet. So please consider carefully whether you are going to use these substances.

On the positive side, exercise has been shown conclusively to increase bone density. Exercise does not have to be strenuous to preserve bone density. Yoga and Tai Chi have been shown to work quite well, although some of my patients would differ whether these are not strenuous!

Regarding supplements for osteoporosis prevention, calcium alone is not adequate. Many of my patients come in with recommendations from their M.D. of 1200 to 1500 mg calcium. At these dosages the body's balance between calcium and magnesium becomes disturbed. I recommend supplemental calcium at 500 to 1000 mg per day. You want calcium citrate or citrate/malate rather than calcium carbonate. The main problem with calcium isn't getting it into your mouth, it's getting it absorbed from the gut into your blood stream. If you don't mind spending more money, microcrystalline hydroxyapatite calcium (or MCHC) has been shown to increase bone mineral density. There are several other minerals that are vital for preserving bone density. These are magnesium, manganese, boron, zinc, and copper. Dosages per day of these are: magnesium at 300 to 600 mg, manganese at 10 to 20 mg, boron at 2 to 3 mg, zinc at 15 to 30 mg, and copper at 2 to 3 mg.

There are also several vitamins that are important in bone metabolism. First among these is vitamin D. The FDA limit of vitamin D is 400 IU, and for most folks this is sufficient, but it is not harmful to take twice this much. In fact, once we reach the age of 55 our absorption of vitamin D drops drastically and many researchers are urging the government to create higher RDA's for folks over 55. Other vitamins for bone include the B vitamins: folic acid at least 800 mcg per day, B6 at least 10 mg, and B12 at least 1000 mcg.

Preliminary findings indicate that the black cohosh extract on the market as Remifemin may be as effective as prescription estrogen replacement therapy at preserving bone mass. Also, many scientists believe the soy isoflavones in tofu and tempeh have this same effect. Please beware of wild yam products marketed as progesterone precursors, as the compounds in this herb need to be transformed by enzymes in the laboratory in order for the progesterone to be available. Look for a statement like "fermented extract" in the ingredient list.

Preventing BPH

Next let's talk about keeping the prostate gland healthy. As I have said previously, the proteins in soy are very beneficial for modulating hormones and keeping the dihydrotestosterone in check, thus preventing BPH. The dose of soy isoflavones is one third of a cake of tofu daily or 500 to 1000 mg of supplemental soy isoflavones. Soy protein powders and soy milk do not have the isoflavones available to us.

Zinc is very important to the prostate gland and may prevent prostate cancer as well as BPH. Adequate doses of zinc are 15 to 30 mg per day.

The amino acids glutamine, alanine, and glycine are good for the prostate. Dosage on these is 300 to 500 mg of each daily. Don't forget that essential fatty acids are vital to the endocrine system. Most of us are deficient in the omega 3's and many of us are deficient in the omega 6's. Some sources of these are flax seeds for the omega 3's, sesame seeds, walnuts, and hemp seeds for a mixture of mainly omega 6's and some omega 3's.

Saw palmetto is rich in phytosterols (plant hormones) and fatty acids that are beneficial for the prostate. Take 150 to 200 mg of saw palmetto extract twice a day.

With that we have reached the end of Tape Five in our series. Thanks for listening and I hope you find this information helpful!

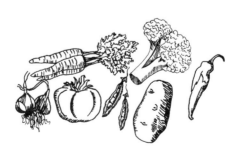

Chapter 6
Danger Drugs

Hello, and welcome to Tape Six of our Free to Be Well© series. On this tape we will be covering Environmental Toxins, Cancer Prevention, and Legal Drugs and their side effects.

Toxic Chemicals & Toxic Metals

First I would like to discuss toxic chemicals. The type of toxic chemicals that I deal with in my practice fall into two main groups. One group is things made by the chemical industry and the second group is toxic metals. Things made by the chemical industry are basically man-made chemicals, things like plastics, herbicides, pesticides, paints and finishes for furniture and wood work, glues, synthetics in clothing and rugs, solvents and strippers, gasoline and petroleum products, lawn and garden chemicals, and household cleaning products. The most common toxic metals that I see causing problems in my patients are aluminum, antimony, arsenic, beryllium, bismuth, cadmium, lead, mercury, silver, tin, and occasionally uranium. I would like to talk about chemicals first and then I will talk about toxic metals.

Toxic Chemicals

Problems with toxic chemicals are usually because of multiple exposures. If I get exposed to a certain pesticide, I do not generally get exposed to enough of it at once (by using it or by eating food farmed with it) that I will get acutely sick. The main problem with all these chemicals is the small doses over long periods of time. These chemicals take a toll on our cells and our liver's ability to take care of its daily burden of toxins. Remember the discussion on Tape Three about liver metabolism? The liver has a certain amount of stuff it has to deal with every day that is made in our body. It also gets exposed to more stuff from outside our body. If the liver cannot keep up with the burden, it has to figure out how it is going to store the backlog of work. The more toxic chemicals that we expose our bodies to, the bigger that backlog gets and the more likely we are to have serious diseases because of the backlog of chemicals.

Toxic Chemical Diseases

The serious diseases caused by these chemicals include cancer, liver diseases, kidney diseases, and neurological diseases like Parkinson's and Multiple Sclerosis. Damage caused by these chemicals starts on a cellular level. They can damage cell membranes, interfering with cell function or killing the cell. Chemicals can damage the genetic material of a cell, predisposing it to becoming the seed of a cancer tumor. One of the most common things chemicals can do is interfere with the ability of our cells to make energy. If we have trouble making energy on a cellular level, then we will feel tired. This can be a potential cause of chronic fatigue syndrome. Another problem that can be caused when chemicals interfere with energy production on a cellular level is fibromyalgia. When muscle cells need to make energy and cannot go about it in the normal way because of a problem in the biochemistry of making energy, they will make energy any way they can. Often the byproducts of this abnormal energy metabolism will cause pain in the muscles that lasts longer than the specific activity. The pain and inflammation from this abnormal energy manufacture often will progress to become fibromyalgia.

I would like to talk a little more specifically about the kinds of damage these chemicals can cause. They can cause liver damage by interfering with the liver's detoxification pathways. Some chemicals may block the Phase I pathway enzymes and other chemicals may block specific Phase II pathways, and in some cases people have become the victims of serious permanent neurological damage or disease because of combined exposure to chemicals that block multiple liver detoxification pathways. Chemicals can interfere with fat metabolism, causing high cholesterol and high triglycerides. At the very least, toxic chemicals can cause the liver cells to store the toxic material because the liver's ability to eliminate it is exceeded. Toxic chemicals also disrupt endocrine metabolism. Many petroleum based compounds (this includes plastics, pesticides, and herbicides) are very similar to estrogens. In women these estrogen-type chemicals can cause or contribute to breast cancer. Many people believe the increased incidence of breast cancer in North America is secondary to the increased environmental exposure of women to these chemicals. Chemicals that are similar to estrogens will cause infertility in men. Many of these compounds will be present in mother's breast milk. Infants and very young children have a decreased ability to deal with these chemicals.

On the cellular level these chemicals can interfere with energy production as we discussed previously. They can also interfere with cell replication. Any time you interfere with the normal ability of cells to reproduce themselves, you create cancerous cells. In a body that is otherwise healthy, the immune system can combat cancer cells effectively, but if the body is overloaded on all fronts by toxic chemicals, then cancer is much more likely to grow and prosper. Last, but certainly not least, many of these chemicals or their byproducts are poisonous to the nervous system. Again, if the liver is overloaded with toxic compounds and things go through the Phase I detox pathways, they become more toxic when they are released into the blood stream than if the liver is able to keep up with its work load and put these chemicals through Phase I and then Phase II. Remember that Phase II is usually the part of the liver's detox pathways that cannot speed up. When you have increased toxic burden to the liver, Phase I will speed up so these toxic compounds go through Phase I. But if Phase II is not ready for them yet, then they get dumped out into the blood stream where they are toxic to both the nervous system and endocrine system.

Exposure to Toxic Chemicals

How do we get exposed to these toxic chemicals? This is going to sound a little simplistic, but the main routes of exposure are: the air we breathe, the water we drink, and the foods we eat. We can also get exposed to them through our skin. As an aside regarding our skin, I am a firm believer that anything we put on our skin should be of the quality that we can eat it because our skin is a living organ. Things we put on our skin are absorbed into our blood stream. We shouldn't put chemicals on our skin that we wouldn't eat. This goes for cosmetics, soaps, and shampoos.

Regarding the air we breathe, if you can smell a chemical in the air then it is present in high enough concentrations to pose a potential burden. The stronger the smell, the higher the dose of that chemical your body is receiving. For example, if you are cleaning your house with bleach and you can smell the bleach, you are getting enough bleach in your lungs that it is getting absorbed into the blood stream. In our modern, industrialized North American society, we get exposed to chemicals on the job, in the air from industry and vehicle exhaust, by lawn and garden chemicals, and the things we use to clean our homes.

Manufactured homes deserve special mention. If you live in a manufactured home you get high doses of chemicals by breathing when you are in your house, for the first two years after the home is manufactured. The chemicals used in the materials of the home "out gas" into the air very heavily when the home is new. I have had more than one patient get very sick after moving into a manufactured home. Chemical doses you breathe in a manufactured home decrease drastically after about two years.

Manufacturing Chemicals

If you live near a manufacturing plant of any kind, you will get chemicals in the air that you breathe. The chemicals that the plant puts out in the air just depend on what they are doing at the factory. Aluminum dust, for example, can travel more than 100 miles in the air from the manufacturing facility. Other toxic metals do not travel quite that far. People who work in the construction industry or who work with paints, solvents, furniture refinishing type chemicals, etc. get exposed to toxic compounds by breathing. There are nontoxic or minimally toxic paints and furniture products on the market as well as nontoxic glues for construction. If you are considering something like installing new carpet, the most toxic part of carpet fumes is the glue that holds it down. Water soluble glues are much less toxic to breathe and work as well as toxic glues. With paints, the toxic compounds in the paints are there to retard spoilage of the paint and extend its shelf life before you buy it. Some manufacturers sell fresh paint that does not need to have all the preservatives and smelly compounds that are also toxic for us to breathe. Ask questions before you buy!

Lawn & Garden Chemicals

Lawn and garden chemicals are a problem through skin exposure and through breathing. If you are using chemicals on your vegetable garden or on your fruit trees, they are a problem because you are eventually going to eat or drink them. I would like to put in a plug here for organic gardening. It is much healthier for people who are going to consume the food and it is also much healthier for the environment. The chemicals we use on our lawn and garden will percolate down through the earth and end up in the water supply.

Drinking Water

There are a variety of things in our drinking water that don't belong in it: toxic metals, chemicals, and microorganisms. Cities tend to test drinking water for certain microorganisms, but many do not test drinking water to make sure it is free of what are called volatile organic chemicals. Those are the gaseous forms of these types of compounds we have been talking about, toxic chemicals from manufacturing and farming. Cities also fail to test municipal water supplies for heavy metals. Believe it or not, there are even certain microorganisms that can be infectious to human beings that most cities do not test the water supply for. Until the public starts asking cities to provide the results of the concentration of these volatile organic chemicals and heavy metals in the water supply, cities are not going to change how they process and filter the water that they are delivering to us.

There are two ways to ensure that drinking water is safe. One way is to get bottled water and the second is to install a filter in your home. I would like to note that bottled water manufacturers are not required to list all the ingredients on the label, so if you are going to use bottled water, it should never taste like plastic. You should not be able to taste the bottle when you drink the water and I would recommend investigating the source of the water and how it is processed to make sure it is actually free of contaminants. Regarding installing a water filter in your home, investigate before you buy a filter. You want to make sure that the filter will eliminate the volatile organic chemicals, heavy metals, and all micro organisms. Some authorities recommend only distilled water or reverse osmosis water. It is my opinion whatever filter you get should eliminate the volatile organics, the heavy metals, and the microorganisms. If so, that water is a vast improvement over what you are probably getting in your municipal water supply.

Foods we Consume

The farming chemicals like herbicides, pesticides, even fertilizers get more concentrated the higher up the food chain we eat. By eating fruits and vegetables, I get a certain dose of these farm chemicals. Animals raised for food like beef, pork, lamb, chicken, etc, will concentrate these agricultural chemicals in their tissues, especially in their fatty tissues. If I eat animals, I get a much higher dose per serving of these chemicals by eating meat and poultry than by eating vegetables. There are some clinicians and scientists who advocate we minimize our exposure to these pesticides by only eating organically raised foods and free-range, organically raised animals. If we can't get vegetables, fruits, grains, and meats that are organically grown or raised, then we should be vegetarians in order to reduce our dose per meal of toxic chemicals in our food.

Prevention

If we have been exposed to these chemicals, and virtually everyone in North America has been exposed to these chemicals at some level, are there certain things we can to do prevent damage caused by these exposures? The answer is yes. The number one thing we can do is to eat a lot of fruits and vegetables. Fruits and vegetables are rich in a variety of compounds that help our body heal its damaged metabolic pathways, and give the liver what it needs to get rid of toxic compounds. Fruits and vegetables are easy for our body to extract nutrition from and fruits provide easily available energy to our cells. In other words they are easy to digest and absorb. I think I have said this on each tape in this series; please eat lots of fruits and vegetables in your diet. Some vegetables that specifically help the body get rid of toxic compounds are the cruciferous family, like broccoli, cauliflower, cabbage, kale, and Brussels sprouts. Vegetables like onions and garlic also contain sulphur. Beets, parsley, and carrots are rich in antioxidants. Don't forget the red-yellow-orange vegetables like tomatoes and squashes. One of the principle herbs that help the liver get rid of toxic compounds is milk thistle also known as Silybum marianum. A healthy daily dose of your principle antioxidants (which includes vitamin C, vitamin E, the carotenoid compounds, the mineral selenium, and lipoic acid) will also help the body minimize damage caused by toxic compounds.

Toxic Metals

The next topic I would like to move on to is toxic metals. The metals I see most commonly in my patients are aluminum, arsenic, antimony, bismuth, cadmium, lead, and mercury. Some of the nutrient minerals can be toxic in high doses. The principle ones in that category are copper, iron, and manganese. These are only toxic if we are exposed to very high doses over long periods of time. Toxic metals are minerals that Mother Nature expected we would get exposed to only in small amounts. In our modern, industrialized society, many of us get exposed to large doses of these metals or minerals and we don't have normal routes to eliminate them. Our body can't use these toxic metals in its normal metabolism. Once we get them in our bodies either in our food or by breathing, then our body has to figure out what to do with them. We strive to get them out of the way. The body says, "This is aluminum, I'm going to store it in bone because it has similar electrical charge to calcium." or similarly, "This is lead and I am going to store it in bone because it has a similar electrical charge to calcium." The body may also try to use the mineral, for example, mercury often will displace selenium in chemical reactions. So the body will try to use the mineral in place of a mineral that has a similar weight or electrical charge. Of course, if an enzyme is dependent on the presence of selenium and mercury gets used in that enzyme, the enzyme is not going to do its job. These toxic heavy metals will interfere with our normal metabolism when they do things like that. When I do hair mineral analysis on my patients, we will often see very high levels of some of these metals like aluminum, cadmium, mercury, lead, etc. People ask me, "How did I get this?" They are thinking of their current exposure. I explain that these tests generally reflect their lifetime history of exposure because the body can't eliminate these toxic metals rapidly so we store them. If they currently cook their food in pots like stainless steel or cast iron and they have high aluminum, but they grew up with food cooked in aluminum pots, then that may be their route of exposure. I have had several patients say to me that they used to play with mercury as kids, that they would use it to make their dimes and quarters shiny or even carry it around in their pockets. Mercury, again, gets absorbed into their body and the body cannot get rid of it, so someone in their 40's can show their childhood exposure to mercury in a hair test today.

Toxic or heavy metals have a variety of poisonous effects on the body. Almost all of them affect the immune system by impairing either white blood cell function or the body's ability to make antibodies. Mercury, in particular, is toxic to the immune system. The same dose of mercury in one person can cause a thousand times more dysfunction in the immune system than the same dose in another person. Cadmium and lead have also been shown to be toxic to the immune system.

Aluminum

Let's talk specifically about some of these metals. Aluminum has been implicated for many years in the development of Alzheimer's disease. There is no question that aluminum exposure causes tangles of neurofibrils in the brain. What has been shown in research on animals is that exposure to aluminum causes more trouble with memory and thinking as the animal gets older. No matter what age the animal was exposed to aluminum, brain function will decline when the animal reaches middle age. Aluminum is also implicated in osteoporosis because the body will also store it in bone, but the main problems with aluminum are memory problems and Alzheimer's type dementia.

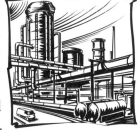

Cadmium

The mineral cadmium is stored in our kidneys primarily and can cause kidney disease and kidney stones. It can also cause osteoporosis. Cadmium damages the liver and causes high blood pressure. Like most of these heavy metals, it is also toxic for the brain and can cause dementia.

Lead

Most of us know that lead is toxic. Lead causes learning and behavior problems in kids and even small amounts of lead will reduce the I.Q. of children. Lead affects children much more than it affects adults. Large amounts of lead can cause dementia and memory problems in adults and trouble with managing anger. Even small amounts of lead in adults have been shown to cause high blood pressure. Lead can also cause anemia. It has an affinity for bones and the gray matter of the brain. Those are the places that the body likes to store it. In general, if I have not mentioned this, the body does not like these toxic metals roaming around in the blood stream indefinitely because all our cells get exposed to their effects. Our body stores these heavy metals in specific locations so they are not traveling all the time.

Mercury

Mercury is probably the most toxic of these metals. Mercury is a very potent neurotoxin. It adversely affects memory, attention span, and concentration. It also can affect mood and can be responsible for depression, irritability, or even suicide. You have probably herd the expression "mad as a hatter." Folks making felt hats historically used mercury to make the hats smooth and shiny and they would eventually go mad because of the absorption of the mercury into their bodies. Mercury can also cause muscle and coordination problems, such as tremors, spasms, and multiple sclerosis. Mercury affects the connective tissue and can be responsible for conditions similar to systemic lupus. Migraine or sinus headaches often respond favorably to the removal of mercury dental fillings. Mercury also affects the heart and can cause chest pain and tachycardia (which is rapid heartbeat). Mercury is toxic to the immune system. If you are like many of my patients who come in saying they do everything they can to boost their immune system, but you have silver-mercury fillings in your teeth this may be the key to improving your immune function. Silver fillings are more than half mercury. The body stores mercury in the liver, kidneys, and brain. In my experience, I see that folks with high mercury have a lot of trouble with the ability of their livers to properly perform detoxification.

Arsenic and Manganese

Arsenic also affects the brain and can cause mood and memory disorders. While it is a nutrient element, manganese in very high levels is problematic. It is associated with antisocial and violent criminal behavior if the body burden of manganese is very high which happens with industrial exposure. Manganese depletes dopamine in the brain and can cause a Parkinson's disease-like syndrome which results in seriously impaired coordination due to destruction of the basal ganglia in the brain.

Aluminum Exposure

You may say that may all be well and good and you haven't been exposed to these metals. Let me clue you in on how we get exposed to these metals and their potential sources. I will first talk about aluminum. For most people the principle routes of aluminum are in the foods and beverages we eat. Foods should not be cooked or stored in aluminum. Acid food like citrus juice or tomatoes will start absorbing significant amounts of aluminum into the food or juice within 20 minutes of exposure. Things like V8 juice or tomato juice that are sold in aluminum cans in the supermarket chelate lots of aluminum into the juice. Please do not drink these juices from aluminum containers. You should never cook tomato sauce in an aluminum pot. Many of the beverages we drink are in aluminum cans, like beer and soda. If you are going to drink these things, please get them in glass bottles as it is the safest material. Don't store food in contact with aluminum foil. Other sources of aluminum are antacids. Many antacids have aluminum in them. All antiperspirants have aluminum. Deodorants generally do not contain aluminum. Check your table salt. Aluminum silicate is an ingredient in table salt to keep it free flowing. Buffered Aspirin, baking powder, pickling salt, and processed cheese are all potential sources of aluminum.

Cadmium Exposure

The majority of my patients with high cadmium have been cigarette smokers, the source that I see most commonly. Other sources for cadmium are black rubber such as tires and carpet backing, water from galvanized pipes, coffee, and evaporated milk. Sewage sludges are generally filled with a lot of toxic metals, but especially cadmium. Fungicides and pesticides have cadmium, and polyvinyl plastics, silver polish, shellfish, and fertilizers also have cadmium.

Lead Exposure

The patients I have seen with high lead exposure generally work in welding or soldering or have other occupational exposure to lead. However, paint in older homes is high in lead. I have seen folks that have been remodeling older homes have high body burdens of lead from breathing the dust of the old paint. Plumbing can be a source of lead in drinking water. Lead is in old newsprint and can be in hair dyes, cable insulation and wire, and also pottery glazes.

Mercury Exposure

Moving on to mercury, the main source of mercury by far is dental fillings. Dental fillings release a significant amount of mercury vapor every time we chew, drink hot liquids, brush our teeth, and even with breathing. We absorb the mercury vapor either directly into the brain through the olfactory nerve at the top of the nasal passage or into the bloodstream from the lungs. Mercury is also used on treated seeds. Skin lightening creams and some medications have mercury. Some paints used to have mercury in them. Seafood can be contaminated by mercury. Polluted water and sewage sludge have mercury in them.

If you ask, your dentist is probably going to tell you that the mercury fillings in your mouth are perfectly safe. I will reiterate that mercury is a very serious toxin. Mercury in the dental office - from the time it arrives in the office until the time they place it in our teeth - has to be treated as a toxic hazard to the folks working in the office. When the silver mercury filling material is removed from our mouths the dental offices again have to treat it as a toxic material. Common sense tells us that mercury filling material is also toxic in our mouths.

I have had several patients with terrible migraine headaches and high mercury on their hair mineral analyses. After following the treatment regimen to help their body eliminate mercury, their headaches resolved almost totally!

How Do we Deal with Toxic Metals?

How do I know whether heavy metals are a problem in my body? Let me explain what I do in my office. If I am suspicious that a patient has symptoms of heavy metal toxicity, I will recommend a hair mineral analysis. If that comes back with high levels of any of the heavy metals, there is a three-prong approach I recommend to my patients. One is that they need to be on baseline nutritional supplementation with multi-minerals, antioxidants, and B-vitamins as we have talked about many times before in this series. The second thing is, I want to put them on a program to insure their liver is doing its detoxification properly. That includes all the dietary things we have talked about like eating a lot of vegetables, especially broccoli, cauliflower, and cabbage, and some nutritional supplements that help the liver do its detox function better. Milk thistle, lipoic acid, and taurine are some examples of things I use in my practice. The third part of the protocol I use to treat these things is chelation.

Chelation is a process where you administer a compound to the body, either orally or intravenously that actually will bind with the toxic substance that the body is having trouble eliminating. The combination of the chelating agent plus the toxic compound, whether it is a metal or chemical, can then be moved out of the body easily by normal metabolic pathways. I put my patients on oral chelation for three months and then retest their hair mineral levels and see whether or not they are improving.

If you are concerned that you may have past or present exposure to these toxic metals, please avoid future exposure and find a practitioner in your area who is willing to test and see whether you have a body burden of these toxic metals presently. If you have silver-mercury amalgam fillings and you chose to get them removed, the best option is to be under the care of a qualified physician who practices natural health care and who is skilled and conversant with detoxification therapies.

Cancer Prevention

The next topic I would like to cover on this tape is cancer prevention. Let's first describe what cancer is. Cancer is any abnormal cell growth. Cancer tumors all start from the abnormal reproduction of normal cells in our bodies. These abnormal cells, changed cells from the original tissues, multiply and grow uncontrollably. The type of tumor depends on which type of cell the cancer started from. Skin cells that become cancerous will be certain types of tumors. Liver or breast cells that become cancerous will develop into other types of tumors. Normally we have cancer cells on and off through our lifetime and our own immune system is able to detect these and destroy them long before detection by science would be possible. We have mechanisms in our immune system that are always seeking out abnormal cells and then calling other forces of the immune system to destroy these abnormal cells. Cancer, in essence, is the failure of our immune system to do its normal job. One of the big problems with cancer is once a tumor has grown large enough to be detected by modern medicine, there is already a very significant underlying problem with that person's metabolism and immune system. They will live under the shadow of that cancer for the rest of their lives, no matter how successful the treatment is.

I would suggest that it is much better to keep our cells healthy and our metabolism happy than to try to fix these things after cancer has started. In my opinion cancer prevention has three main aspects. The first one that all of us should be familiar with is minimizing or eliminating the exposure to things that can actually cause cancer. These are toxic chemicals, heavy metals, and some substances in our food supply. The second part of this is a basic healthy diet and nutritional supplement program. In other words, give our cells what they need to do their job properly, and when it is time for them to go through cellular division, everything will be there that they need to do that normally and they will not produce abnormal cells — we hope. The third part of cancer prevention in my opinion is making sure that the GI tract — the gut and liver — are doing their jobs properly. We want a normal, healthy environment in the colon, and the liver providing the proper detoxification function in the body. There are many folks in natural health care that say one of the cardinal rules regarding cancer is keeping the digestive tract healthy.

Carcinogens

We already talked on the beginning of this tape about toxic chemicals that are present in our industrialized society. They include household, industrial, agricultural, and gardening chemicals. You can feel free to consider any or all of the above as carcinogenic, that is, things that can cause cancer. Many of the toxic metals we just talked about in the last topic are carcinogens given the right conditions.

The last category of carcinogens we have not yet talked about are things that are normally part of our food supply. The most problematic of these potential carcinogens is polyunsaturated vegetable oils. The polyunsaturated oils are extremely reactive and will react with whatever is close at hand. When we eat them, they are likely to react with our own cell membranes, our own enzymes, or whatever else is close at hand for them to react with inside our bodies. Please do not believe all the advertising hype about corn oil products, hydrogenated or partially hydrogenated vegetable oil products, being more healthy for your heart and blood vessels. The truth is, they are not healthy for your heart or blood vessels and they are also carcinogenic. The fats to avoid here are polyunsaturated vegetable oils and partially hydrogenated and hydrogenated vegetable oils (corn oil, soy oil, margarine, processed foods, etc.) Deep frying creates similar carcinogenic compounds in the oil. Fried foods should be avoided as well.

Processed meats like lunch meats, sausage, bacon, and ham are particularly carcinogenic because of the added nitrites. Nitrites cause cancer in test animals at a fraction of the concentration present in the meats people eat. Please check labels for food additives. These chemicals are added to our food in small amounts for whatever reason. They may be added as flavorings, colorings, or preservatives. Many of these compounds are also potential carcinogens.

The effects of multiple chemical residues in our foods, whether it is things that are intentionally added to our food (like preservatives, flavorings, and colorings), or things that are in the food because of the agricultural business (like herbicides, pesticides, and fertilizer residues) is totally unknown. Single compounds have been tested for their effects in human beings, but the combination of these compounds end up being a chemical soup that nobody has tested. No one knows how this chemical soup affects our immune system, cells, or genetic material. There is evidence if there is more than one chemical in a food that the effects of the chemicals together do not add one to another, they actually multiply each other. The safest thing if we care about our health, is to absolutely minimize the amount of chemicals we get in our diet.

I would also be remiss if I didn't mention that cigarette smoking and cigarette smoke is a causative agent in a variety of cancers. If you smoke and want to prevent cancer in yourself and your loved ones, please figure out a way to quit!

Dietary Cancer Prevention

So, now we've eliminated toxins from our diet and as much as possible from our exposure, so we are not using toxic chemicals to clean our house, in our yard, etc. The first thing on the positive side of cancer prevention is the type of things we have talked about on previous tapes; eating a good healthy diet that will support our normal cellular function. Again, many of the phytonutrients that are continually being discovered in fruits and vegetables have active compounds in them that support normal cellular function and enable our body to fight cancer and the damage caused by daily wear and tear. Please eat your vegetables and your fruits and eat a lot of them every day!

Remember I said on the first tape that I like people to get at least two cups of vegetables per day. Four cups would be even better. That is the non-starchy vegetables, so white potatoes do not count as a vegetable. If you are going to add fat to your vegetables, keep it to a minimum and please remember, no bad fats. One idea a patient told me about, which I thought was great, was adding fresh flaxseed oil over her vegetables after they were cooked. That got her the essential fatty acids along with the good nutrients in the vegetables.

Nutritional Supplementation
to Support Cancer Prevention

As far as nutritional supplements for preventing cancer, the number one category of nutritional supplements is going to be your antioxidants. There is a lot of scientific data supporting antioxidants' preventive effects on the development of cancer tumors. The other class of nutritional supplements that I keep seeing in the literature I read is the sulfur bearing amino acids and other sulphur compounds. Some antioxidants are: beta-carotene and vitamin A, vitamin C, vitamin E, selenium, and lipoic acid. The sulfur bearing compounds that help improve liver detox function and are also being shown to prevent cancer are things like reduced glutathione, methionine, taurine, and a supplement known by the initials MSM which stands for methylsulphonylmethane. Of course the broccoli, cauliflower, cabbage, Brussels sprouts, kale family of vegetables are high in sulfur. Onions and garlic are also high in sulfur compounds. I also strongly recommend a basic foundation of multi-vitamins. A body needs calcium, magnesium, chromium, zinc, copper, boron, manganese — all of these minerals are very important. Each of the B-vitamins are vital for proper cellular function.

The next recommendation for preventing cancer is keep the liver and GI system healthy. I have talked about both of those at length on Tape Two and Tape Three, so I will not take up any more space on this tape for those subjects.

Prescription Drugs

The last topic I would like to cover on this tape is side effects of prescription drugs and over the counter medications. I would like to introduce this by saying that if you are taking a prescription medication for any reason, **do not** take the information on this tape to mean you should not be taking your specific medication. You need to have a qualified clinician evaluate your specific health condition to help you decide whether or not you should be taking a medication that has been prescribed for you. The information I am giving here is for people who are deciding whether or not to start a prescription medication. If you are in that situation, if any of the information that I have to say here strikes a resonant cord with you, please talk it over with the clinician who will be prescribing the medication for you. Please do not use the information on this tape to make an uninformed decision about whether or not you specifically need medications.

Some of the most commonly prescribed medications that my patients come in already taking are medications controlling blood pressure, antidepressants (Prozac, Effexor, Paxil, and Zoloft), Premarin or other hormone replacement therapies, cholesterol lowering drugs

(Mevacor, Lovistatin), antibiotics, and corticosteroid medications like Prednisone. In my practice, one of the first things I do when I am trying to figure out why a patient has certain symptoms is to look at the side effects of the drugs they are taking. Often the symptoms a patient comes in complaining of are listed in the technical literature about the patient's medication as side effects. It is well known in the drug business that for every prescription drug a patient is taking, that individual will need two more medications to deal with the side effects from the first drug that they were prescribed.

Antibiotic Medications

Of all the drugs that I have mentioned on this list, I would like to pick on antibiotics and Prednisone first because in my practice these are the ones that seem to cause the most long-term problems associated with their side effects. We have talked quite a bit about antibiotics and side effects of antibiotics on Tape Two with the GI system. The typical worst case scenarios that I see after antibiotic use are adults who had antibiotics many, many times as children. Somewhere during adolescence or young adulthood, they started developing the kinds of chronic health problems that most of us would hope to never experience until we become elderly. These may be things like fibromyalgia, chronic fatigue syndrome, and arthritis in multiple joints. The typical person who comes to me with this kind of scenario usually has a Candida infection, and the Candida is usually systemic. If we test their blood, we can find antibodies to the Candida in their blood stream. The reason antibiotics predispose people to Candida infection is that antibiotics are fairly effective at killing bacteria including the beneficial bacteria lining the colon, but antibiotics do not kill fungi. We normally have very small amounts of Candida in our large intestines. When you kill off the bacteria lining the large intestine, then you set up this wonderful environment for the Candida to grow on the nice, wet, soft, colonic membrane. So instead of having the beneficial bacteria against the wall of the colon, you now have a lot of colonies of yeast growing and some of the little yeast cells will get absorbed into the blood stream and they can set up housekeeping in the spleen, liver, or whatever.

Studies have shown that antibiotics do not improve the outcome in kids with ear infections, and recommendations to M.D. pediatricians are against the use of antibiotics for kids with ear infections.

Prednisone

Prednisone is another drug that predisposes people to yeast infections. Prednisone is given to suppress our normal immune function. When it does this, it makes it much more easy for us to get Candida infections. Infections are a common side effect of corticosteroid therapy.

However, most of the problems with corticosteroids including Prednisone have to do with long-term use of the drug. As we saw in Tape Five, that includes diabetes. These drugs also cause debilitating osteoporosis over the long term. They can cause high blood pressure. Remember from Tape Five we talked about the muscle wasting that happens with corticosteroids, so they will cause muscle weakness and changes in the distribution of the fat in the body. We have fat pads in our feet to cushion the bones in our feet when we walk. Long term use can cause the disappearance of those fat pads which can cause foot pain.

Cholesterol Medications

The next category of drugs that I am going to talk about is the new cholesterol lowering drugs. The cholesterol lowering drugs that bother me and worry me the most when people come in taking them are in the class of the HMG Co A Reductase inhibitors. This HMG Co A Reductase is an enzyme in the liver, and it acts in the cholesterol pathway. If you remember, on tape five we talked about the importance of cholesterol to the endocrine system. That discussion provides insight into why people in the nutritional field are so worried about these drugs. When you inhibit these enzymes, you will inhibit the body's ability to make hormones normally. Nobody really knows what the effect of a drug like this can be in any given patient, or what the effects of a drug like this will be when they are used long term in large groups of people. The names of these drugs are Lovistatin, also known as Mevacor, Pravostatin, also known as Pravocol, and Symbistatin, also known as Zocor. The most common problem with these drugs is liver damage, and patients who are taking these drugs should have periodic blood tests. I like my patients on these drugs to get a complete panel of liver enzymes, that is five different enzymes, checked every six months. These drugs can also cause muscle and chest pain, they can cause nausea, diarrhea, headaches, abdominal gas, and muscle breakdown. I have seen patients with serious endocrine (both adrenal and thyroid) problems secondary to taking these drugs.

The other main class of cholesterol lowering drugs are resins that bind with bile acids. The liver excretes cholesterol in the bile. If you take these drugs orally, they do not get absorbed into the blood stream, but they bind with bile acid in the intestines. They hold cholesterol in the large intestine, normally cholesterol gets reabsorbed from the large intestine to participate in hormone cycles. If it is not getting reabsorbed, then these drugs will actually cause the liver to make more cholesterol than it was making. These drugs' names are Questran and Cholested and they will also interfere with fat metabolism and the absorption of fat and fat soluble vitamins from the gut. They can cause constipation as well. These drugs can also be problematic for the liver, and liver enzymes should be tested at least every six months if you are taking these drugs.

Antidepressants

Next on my list of pet peeves in the prescription drug department are the antidepressants, the new serotonin reuptake inhibitors, like Prozac, Effexor, and Zoloft. Two of the common side effects that I see in my practice secondary to these medications are musculoskeletal pain, generally aching pain around the spine and the large joints like the shoulders and hips. The other side effect that I have seen secondary to these medications is belly pain. I have seen patients with stomach pain that was absolutely incapacitating. I have one patient who has ended up in the emergency room more than once after just a short course of one of these medications. She discontinued it because the belly pain was so bad she was incapacitated. I have seen other patients with ongoing belly pain get evaluated with all the sophisticated medical testing and have no physical problem with their stomach, small intestine, or gall bladder. It turns out the antidepressant is causing their discomfort and pain.

The other problem that I have seen in my practice with these drugs is that once people start them, because of their effect on the central nervous system, they have a much more difficult time with their depression if they try to stop the drug. I have seen people become suicidal when they try to stop these drugs. If you want to discontinue one of these medications, you must be under the supervision of a physician.

Another concern that I have about antidepressants has been expressed by other folks in the health care field. With our current health insurance system, many HMO's are more willing to pay for prescriptions for these medications than they are to pay for psychotherapy or counseling. In the long run, the effects of the psychotherapy or counseling in an individual person's life is much more beneficial than being on Prozac indefinitely.

Hormone Replacement Therapy

The single most commonly prescribed medication is Premarin. Premarin is primarily horse estrogens. I have seen all kinds of side effects secondary to Premarin or other prescription hormone replacement medications. Many women who take them are very uncomfortable on these medications. As we said on Tape Five, it can predispose people to adult onset diabetes, blood clots, and stroke. Some of the side effects that I have seen from these medications in my office are dizziness, nausea, and very painful esophageal spasms, with difficulty swallowing.

The primary reason for so many side effects with these hormone replacements is that the compounds are not the same estrogens or progesterones that occur naturally in our bodies. Prescription progesterone is Medroxyprogesterone which is synthetic and is only vaguely similar to the progesterone that occurs in women's bodies. The estrogens that are used are either synthetic or mainly estradiol. Women do have estradiol, but it is 10% or less of human circulating estrogens. The predominant estrogen in women is estriol which is 80-90% of the total circulating estrogen in women. The effects of estriol are still being studied.

It is suspected that estriol is actually protective against breast cancer. I neglected to mention that one of the side effects of estrogen replacement therapies is breast cancer. That, again, is because of the synthetic estrogens and the overload of estradiol. What happens with these prescription estrogens is that it takes the liver in some cases 2000 times longer to break these down. These potent estrogens are circulating in the blood stream, stimulating estrogen receptors in breast and uterine tissue. This results in over stimulation of these tissues. That is thought to be the mechanism for cancer development secondary to these drugs.

Blood Pressure Medications

The last class of prescription drugs that I want to talk about is blood pressure medications. The use of blood pressure medications in people with mild to moderate hypertension is controversial within the medical community and it is well known that most patients, when they are put on blood pressure medications, are much more uncomfortable on the medication than off the medication. In my practice I have seen more than one patient who did not materially improve on these drugs. I will caution you again, you cannot abruptly discontinue a blood pressure medication. Please do not construe the information on this tape to be advocating you stop these drugs.

The first line blood pressure medications are diuretics which help the body eliminate fluids. The side effects with these are loss of potassium and/or magnesium. There is also risk of heart attack or stroke with these drugs because they are more likely to cause blood clots. They often will increase cholesterol and triglycerides which is not something you want to see in someone with high blood pressure. They can also cause low blood pressure and light-headedness.

The beta blockers, drugs like Lopressor and Inderal can cause people to be foggy headed, tired, dizzy, and depressed. These drugs will also raise cholesterol and triglycerides.

Calcium channel blockers, drugs like Cardiogram, Cardene, and Procardia can cause fluid retention, dizziness, headache, fatigue, constipation, and occasionally chest pain.

ACE inhibitors, are the "prils", drugs like Acupril, Captopril, Vasotec, and Zestril. These drugs cause potassium retention which can, in some cases, lead to heart problems and kidney problems. In some folks they may also cause dizziness, light-headedness, headache, or the development of a cough during the night. Because of the "prils'" effect on the kidneys, a decrease in dosage will cause a rebound of blood pressure. Do not stop taking a "pril" if you are on one of these without consulting your clinician.

Over-the-Counter Medications

Next we will talk about over-the-counter medications. The most common over-the-counter medications that my patients come in taking are ibuprofen products like Advil and Motrin. Other types of pain medications like Tylenol, and digestive aids like Tagamet and Pepcid are also common. Of these drugs I have listed, ibuprofen is probably the least problem. Ibuprofen is only a serious problem for people who have kidney disease. People with kidney disease should know not to take ibuprofen. Tylenol, Tagamet, and Pepcid all interfere with normal liver detox pathways and Tylenol can be lethal when combined with alcohol use. Regarding Tylenol, some people who take it on a daily basis with alcohol like wine or beer will actually kill the liver over time. The only remedy compatible with survival is a liver transplant.

Tylenol, Tagamet, or Pepcid in combination with inhaled lawn or garden chemicals can cause permanent neurological damage or death.

With that I have come to the end of my material for this tape. Thanks for hanging in there for our entire series, and I hope you have found this program informative!

Some Closing Reminders

The basics of staying healthy are fairly simple. Eat foods as close to their natural state as possible. For example, steamed or sauteed fresh organic vegetables are more nutritious and richer in antioxidant compounds than canned vegetables grown with herbicides and pesticides. Whole grain foods are more nutritious and healthier for your digestive tract than refined white flour products. Avoid products from animals who have been fed antibiotics or hormones. Remember, Mom always said to eat your vegetables. Two to four cups of vegetables daily will provide your body with a rich variety of bioflavonoids and other antioxidant compounds. There is no better way to make your cells happy!

Get in the habit of reading the ingredient labels on the foods you buy. If an ingredient doesn't seem like food, it probably isn't. Your body will thank you for not eating it! Don't eat toxic fats like hydrogenated oils or refined polyunsaturated vegetable oils. Do eat good quality fats like fresh fish, fresh nuts, and seeds. Eat as little sugar, sweets, and alcohol as possible. None is best! Keep your liver happy, minimize your exposure to chemicals and toxic metals.

Our cells can't be happy if the ecosystem in the intestines is out of balance. Everything we put in our mouths affects the delicate balance of microbes in the gut. Try to think of eating as a way to grow a healthy garden in the colon. Remember, microbes are going to be there, if we don't feed the good bugs, then the bad bugs will predominate.

Make a habit of taking a good quality multivitamin-mineral daily. But, remember that no vitamins or supplements can make up for a poor quality diet. We are what we eat. Eat well in health!

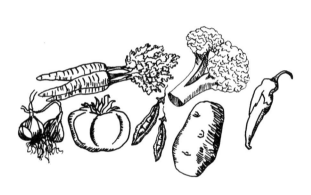

Glossary of Terms

acidophilus: a species of beneficial bacteria in the colon

adrenal: an endocrine gland that sits on top of the kidney

adrenalin: one of the "fight or flight" hormones made by the adrenal glands

alanine: an amino acid, one of the building blocks of protein

albumin: a protein prevalent in the blood stream

alcoholism: disease of alcohol addiction

aldosterone: a hormone made by the adrenal glands

Alzheimer's disease: a degenerative disease of the brain involving loss of memory and thinking abilities

amino acids: building blocks from which proteins are made

amylase: an enzyme that digests starch, present in saliva and made by the pancreas

androgens: "male" hormones

anti-inflammatory: any compound or metabolic pathway that decreases cellular irritation

anti-microbial: any substance or metabolic pathway toxic to foreign "bugs" (bacteria, viruses, yeasts, etc.)

anti-oxidants: compounds that prevent damage to cells and cell membranes caused by oxygen free radicals

antibiotic: a drug that kills bacteria

antibodies: proteins made by the immune system specifically to initiate the attack of foreign proteins

asthma: a disease of the large airways of the lungs

atherosclerosis: hardening of the arteries

bacteria: a class of single celled organisms

beta-carotene: a precursor of vitamin A, present in many vegetables

bifidobacter: a species of beneficial bacteria in the colon

bile: a substance made in the liver, collected and concentrated in the gall bladder, and excreted into the small intestine to aid with fat digestion

bromelain: an enzyme present in pineapple that breaks down protein, used as an anti-inflammatory or to aid digestion

Candida: a species of yeast normally present in small amounts in the colon

candidiasis: overgrowth of Candida which causes a variety of
    symptoms

carnitine: an amino acid, one of the building blocks of protein

carotenoids: a class of anti-oxidant compounds, one of which is
    beta-carotene

cataract: opacity in the lens of the eye

cell receptors: locations on cell membranes waiting to combine
    with specific hormones and initiate a response inside the cell

cellulase: an enzyme which aids in breakdown of cellulose

chasteberry: an herb used to balance female hormones

chelation: use of a compound to bind with unwanted toxins and
    hold the toxins in a form the body can eliminate

chronic fatigue syndrome: a condition of long term fatigue,
    sometimes associated with Epstein-Bar virus and/or depression

colitis: inflammation of the lining of the large intestine

colon: the large intestine

congestive heart failure: a disease in which heart muscle strength
    gradually fails

CoQ-10: an enzyme that aids in energy production by cells

corticosteroids: drugs used to suppress the immune system, or
    hormones made naturally by the adrenal glands

cortisol: hormone made by the adrenal glands which plays a role
    in managing blood sugar and immune function

cysteine: an amino acid, one of the building blocks of protein

delayed food allergies: immune reactions to ingested foods that
    cause symptoms between 6 hours and 3 days after eating the
    food

dermatitis: an inflammatory condition of the skin

detoxification: metabolic process of changing toxins so they can
    be easily excreted

DHEA: dehydroepiandrosterone, a hormone made by the adrenal
    glands

diabetes: a disease whose principle feature is loss of control of blood
    sugar levels

digestive enzymes: enzymes that aid in breaking down foods we eat

digestive tract: esophagus, stomach, and intestines

diuretics: herbs or medications that promote excretion of water by the kidneys

dopamine: a hormone made by the brain and by the adrenal glands

dysmenorrhea: difficult menstruation, usual symptoms are heavy cramping, heavy bleeding, low back pain, nausea, or vomiting

endocrine glands: organs in the body that make hormones and secrete them into the blood stream

enzymes: proteins that initiate chemical reactions

ephedra: a stimulant herb which can cause heart rhythm disturbances or heart attacks

epinephrine: one of the "fight or flight" hormones made by the adrenal glands

estradiol: a type of estrogen

estrogen: a "female" hormone

estrogenic herbs: herbs that stimulate estrogen receptors of cells

fibromyalgia: a disease involving muscle pain and fatigue

folic acid: a B vitamin

FOS: fructo-oligosaccharides, a type of fiber that nourishes beneficial
    gut bacteria

fungi: mushrooms and yeasts

fungicides: compounds that kill fungi

gall bladder: organ nestled under the liver that collects bile from the liver and excretes it into the small intestine

gastrointestinal system: the digestive system, stomach, intestines, liver, gall bladder, and pancreas

GI tract: gastrointestinal tract

globulin: a variety of large proteins in the blood stream, some transport hormones, others participate in allergic reactions

glucagon: a hormone secreted by the pancreas that maintains blood sugar levels between meals

glutamine: an amino acid, one of the building blocks of protein

glutathione: an amino acid, one of the building blocks of protein

glycemic index: measure of how much a specific food raises blood sugar

glycine: an amino acid, one of the building blocks of protein

glycogen: form in which the muscle cells and liver store sugar for energy production

gout: a type of arthritis

H2 blockers: a class of drugs used for stomach pain

HDL: high density lipoprotein, the "good" cholesterol

hepatitis: inflammation of the liver, usually an infectious viral disease

homocysteine: a byproduct of inflammatory metabolism in the presence of B-vitamin deficiencies

hydrochloric acid: acid form present in the stomach

hypoallergenic diet: a diet which eliminates all of the common allergy-causing foods

hypoglycemia: low blood sugar

insulin: a hormone made by the pancreas and secreted into the blood stream to move sugar from the blood into the cells

insulin resistance: a condition in which the cells become unresponsive to insulin in the blood stream causing insulin levels to rise to maintain normal blood sugar levels

intestinal permeability: inflammation of the lining of the intestines which allows exposure of the blood stream to intestinal contents

l-glutamine: an amino acid, one of the building blocks of protein

LDL: low density lipoprotein, one type of "bad" cholesterol

leaky gut syndrome: condition in which the intestinal lining is inflamed and exposes the blood stream to the gut contents

lipase: enzyme that breaks down fat

lipoic acid: a potent antioxidant vitamin

lithium: a nutrient mineral

liver: large solid organ below the right diaphragm, makes bile; is responsible for carbohydrate, fat, and protein metabolism; plays a significant part in immune function and removal of toxins

liver detox pathway: complex reactions the liver uses to change substances in the blood stream to nontoxic forms that can be excreted easily

lymphatic system: a system of vessels throughout the body that collects pooled fluid from between cells and returns it to the blood stream

mal-absorption: condition in which nutrients are not absorbed from the intestines into the blood stream

methionine: an amino acid, one of the building blocks of protein

milk thistle: an herb which aids in liver function

mitochondria: organelles (tiny organs) inside each of our cells responsible for making energy

monounsaturated: fat molecule which has one carbon-carbon double bond available

MSM: methylsulphonylmethane, a supplemental form of sulfur

mucosa: specialized cells that produce protective mucus

mucosal lining: specialized mucus producing cells lining the respiratory, digestive, and genitourinary tracts

multiple sclerosis: a progressive disease of the brain and spinal cord; usual symptoms include loss of coordination, balance, and/or muscle control, impaired vision is common

neurofibrils: tangles of connective tissue that grow in the brain and interfere with its ability to do its job

neurotoxin: anything that poisons nerve cells of the brain, spinal cord, or body

niacin: vitamin B3

nightshade family: plant relatives of tobacco, tomato, and potato

omega 3: class of essential fatty acids

omega 6: class of essential fatty acids

organophosphate compounds: chemical neurotoxins, commonly used in insecticides

osteoporosis: condition in which bone loses density and becomes brittle

ovaries: paired glands in women that produce eggs

oxidation: damage caused by reactive forms of oxygen

P450 enzymes: enzymes used by Phase I detox pathways

pancreas: an organ which makes hormones to regulate blood sugar and enzymes to aid digestion

pancreatic enzymes: enzymes secreted into the small intestine by the pancreas to aid in digestion

pantethine: the active form of vitamin B5

Parkinson's disease: a disease of the basal ganglia of the brain in which coordination deteriorates

pepsin: a digestive factor produced in the stomach to aid the breakdown of protein

phosphatidyl choline: a B vitamin especially beneficial to cell membranes

phosphatidyl inositol: a B vitamin especially beneficial to cell membranes

pituitary: "the master gland", located just under the brain, it makes several hormones that tell other glands how much to produce

Prednisone: a synthetic drug version of adrenal cortisol

Premarin: a drug form of estrogen derived from horse urine

proanthocyanadin: a type of antioxidant nutrient

probiotics: beneficial gut bacteria used as supplements

progesterogenic herbs: herbs that stimulate progesterone receptors

progesterone: a "female" hormone

prostaglandins: compounds made by white blood cells, some cause inflammation and some relieve inflammation

prostate: a gland in men that surrounds the urethra

protease: an enzyme that breaks down protein

pycnogenol: an antioxidant nutrient

pyridoxal 5' phosphate: the active form of vitamin B6

quercitin: a nutrient in the bioflavonoid class

quinoa: a grain which is high in protein and free of gluten

relaxin: a hormone secreted during pregnancy which loosens mom's ligaments to allow an easier birth

riboflavin 5' phosphate: the active form of vitamin B2

saliva: also know as spit (the noun)

selenium: an antioxidant mineral

somatostatin: a hormone that inhibits release of growth hormone

soy isoflavones: phytosterols or plant hormones naturally present in soy

taurine: an amino acid, one of the building blocks of protein

tempeh: a fermented soybean cake

testosterone: a "male" hormone

thyroglobulin: the carrier protein for thyroid hormone

thyroid: a gland responsible for metabolic rate

thyroxine: thyroid hormone

tofu: curd made from soybean milk

triglycerides: long chain fat molecules

tyrosine: an amino acid, one of the building blocks of protein

urethra: tube through which urine leaves the bladder

uterus: womb

viruses: organisms consisting only of genetic material and a protein coat that must use living cells in order to reproduce

VLDL: very low density lipoprotein, most damaging subtype of cholesterol

Questions and Answers

The following are questions raised by my editor as she read the manuscript of Free to Be Well$^©$. Because the master CD for the tapes is finished, this information had to be included as an appendix rather than as a change to the text of the respective chapters.

Happy Hearts:

Q: Why doesn't the high density (HDL) cholesterol stop moving? Aren't heavier things harder to keep moving than lighter things?

A: The heavier cholesterol has a higher proportion of protein to lipid, is more compact, and more slippery in the blood stream. The lipids of LDL and VLDL cholesterols are much more easily oxidized, and in their oxidized forms are very sticky.

Q: When cholesterol levels rise on very low fat diets, why don't both LDL and HDL levels rise?

A: The liver needs an array of nutrients to produce HDL (good cholesterol). Essential fatty acids are necessary for the production of HDL; these are too often absent in low fat diets, hence the rise in LDL only.

Q: Why do margarine and other hydrogenated fats lower HDL cholesterol?

A: Again, with these fats in the diet, folks are usually deficient in the omega 3 essential fatty acids needed for HDL production.

Q: Why does oxidation of LDL damage blood vessel walls?

A: Oxidized molecules are highly reactive, oxidized LDL reacts with blood vessel membranes and impairs membrane integrity.

Q: Why is hydrogenated fat, like margarine, bad if saturated fat isn't?

A: Hydrogenated fat has been made toxic by the extreme heat and harsh chemicals applied to vegetable oils in the refining and hydrogenation processes. Hydrogenated fat accelerates inflammation and damages cell membranes.

Q: What does insoluble fiber do in the diet?

A: Insoluble fiber provides bulk to stool by holding water in the colon. Some types of insoluble fiber also provide a growth media for beneficial bacteria.

Leaping Livers

Q: Which is doing the detoxification, the enzymes or the phase pathway?

A: The Phase I pathways are mainly reactions which use the P450 enzymes. So, in Phase I, these enzyme reactions *are* the detox pathway. However, in Phase II, the detoxification is performed by other compounds.

Q: Does Phase I render compounds more toxic than before?

A: Yes, some compounds are far more toxic after Phase I than before. These compounds need to go through Phase II, as well, in order to be rendered nontoxic.

Q: Why are drugs like Tagamet, Pepcid, and Tylenol bothersome?

A: Each of these drugs completely block one of the Phase II detox pathways preventing other toxic compounds from being rendered non-toxic by the same pathway.

Demystifying Diets

Q: You mention symptoms foods may cause on a Candida diet, but you don't say what they are.

A: Foods that promote growth of Candida are different for each person. Symptoms may include: joint or muscle pain, fatigue, bloating, sore throat or tongue, skin rashes, athlete's foot, etc.

Glad Glands

Q: What is the difference between hormones and enzymes?

A: Enzymes catalyze or initiate reactions between compounds whenever they encounter the biochemicals they are keyed to react with. Hormones are made by one organ to act on a cell receptor in a different organ or tissue. Hormones travel through the blood stream without causing any changes until they arrive at the target tissue.

Q: Why is a diet low in sweets, alcohol, and refined starches better for the pancreas?

A: All of these foods cause large and rapid elevations of blood sugar. Rapid spikes of blood sugar call on the pancreas to produce insulin rapidly. If the pancreas is called on to produce lots of insulin frequently, it may get tired and unable to produce adequate insulin. This allows blood sugar to remain elevated causing diabetes.

Q: Do cortisol and glucagon work together to maintain fasting blood sugar?

A: Yes.

Q: Why do moms become progressively more deficient in essential fatty acids with each pregnancy?

A: Because most of us do not eat nearly enough essential fatty acids in our diet and mom's body will give the baby what it needs to grow at mom's expense. The mother's existing reservoirs of essential fatty acids go to her baby, and are shrunk more by each succeeding pregnancy.

Q: What is the difference between soy proteins and soy isoflavones?

A: Soy protein is any protein present in soy. Soy isoflavones are the phytosterols, or plant hormones, naturally present in soy foods. These isoflavones are most available in tofu and tempeh.

Danger Drugs

Q: Why is depletion of dopamine a problem in manganese toxicity? What does dopamine do?

A: Dopamine is one of the hormones used by the nervous system, including the brain, to communicate between nerve cells. Depletion of dopamine interferes with communication between nerve cells.

Q: Which food additives are potential carcinogens?

A: Possible carcinogenic compounds in food include: synthetic dyes, preservatives, synthetic flavorings, nitrites, bad fats, as well as residues of antibiotics, hormones, herbicides, pesticides, heavy metals, and other toxins commonly used in farming.

References

Chapter 1 ♡ Happy Hearts

Alderman JD, Pasternak RC, et al. Effect of a modified, well-tolerated niacin regimen on serum total cholesterol, high density lipoprotein cholesterol and the cholesterol to high density lipoprotein ratio. *Am J Cardiol* 1989 Oct 1;64(12):725-9.

Anderson JW. Dietary fibre, complex carbohydrate and coronary artery disease. *Can J Cardiol* 1995; 11 Suppl G: 55G-62G.

Anderson JW, Hanna TJ. Impact of Nondigestible Carbohydrates on Serum Lipoproteins and Risk for Cardiovascular Disease. *J Nutr* 1999; 129(7 Suppl): 1457S-1466S.

Anderson JW, Johnstone BM, Cook-Newell ME. Meta-analysis of the effects of soy protein intake on serum lipids. *N Engl J Med* 1995; 333(5): 276-82.

Ascherio A, Willett WC. Health effects of trans fatty acids. *Am J Clin Nutr* 1997; 66(4 Suppl): 1006S-1010S.

Bergomi M, Rovesti S, et al. Zinc and copper status and blood pressure. *J Trace Elem Med Biol* 1997 Nov;11(3):166-9.

Bushehri N, Jarrell ST et al. Oral reduced B-nicotinamide adenine dinucleotide (NADH) affects blood pressure, lipid peroxidation, and lipid profile in hypertensive rats (SHR). *Geriatr Nephrol Urol* 1998; 8(2): 95-100.

Davey PJ, Schulz M et al. Cost-effectiveness of vitamin E therapy in the treatment of patients with angiographically proven coronary narrowing (CHAOS trail). Cambridge Heart Antioxidant Study. *Am J Cardiol* 1998; 82(4): 414-7.

Dubick MA, Keen CL, et al. Antioxidant enzyme activity in human abdominal aortic aneurysmal and occlusive disease. *Proc Soc Exp Biol Med* 1999 Jan;220(1):39-45.

Figge HL, Figge J, et al. Nicotinic acid: a review of its clinical use in the treatment of lipid disorders. *Pharmacotherapy* 1988;8(5):287-294.

Forsythe WA, Green MS, Anderson JJ. Dietary protein effects on cholesterol and lipoprotein concentrations: a review. *J Am Coll Nutr* 1986;5(6):533-49.

Gondal JA, MacArthy P et al. Effects of dietary sucrose and fibers on blood pressure in hypertensive rats. *Clin Nephrol* 1996; 45(3): 163-8.

Guallar E, Aro A et al. Omega-3 fatty acids in adipose tissue and risk of myocardial infarction: the EURAMIC study. *Arterioscler Thromb Vasc Biol* 1999; 19(4): 1111-8.

Kagan VE, Serbinova EA, et al. Recycling of vitamin E in human low density lipoproteins. *J Lipid Res* 1992 Mar;33(3):385-97.

Kinlay S, Fang JC, et al. Plasma alpha-tocopherol and coronary endothelium-dependent vasodilator function. *Circulation* 1999 Jul 20;100(3):219-21.

Kugiyama K, Motoyama T et al. Improvement of endothelial vasomotor dysfunction by treatment with alpha-tocopherol in patients with high remnant lipoproteins levels. *J Am Coll Cardiol* 1999; 33(6): 1512-8.

Lichtenstein AH, Ausman LM, et al. Effects of different forms of dietary hydrogenated fats on serum lipoprotein cholesterol levels. *N Eng J Med* 1999 Jun 24;340(25):1933-40.

Manson JE, Bronner LL, Kanter DS. Primary prevention of stroke. *N Engl J Med* 1995; 333:1392-1400.

Mohan JC, Arora R, Khalilullah M. Preliminary observations on effect of Lactobacillus sporogenes on serum lipid levels in hypercholesterolemic patients. *Indian J Med Res* 1990 Dec;92:431-2.

Mori TA, Beilin LJ, et al. Interactions between dietary fat, fish, and fish oils and their effects on platelet function in men at risk of cardiovascular disease. *Arterioscler Thromb Vasc Biol* 1997 Feb;17(2):279-86.

Nyyssonen K, Parviainen MT et al. Vitamin C deficiency and risk of myocardial infarction: prospective population study of men from eastern Finland. *BMJ* 1997; 314(7981): 634-8.

O'Keefe JH Jr, Harris WS, et al. Effects of pravastatin with niacin or magnesium on lipid levels and postprandial lipemia. *Am J Cardiol* 1995 Sep 1;76(7):489-4.

Ozer NK, Sirikci O, et al. Effect of vitamin E and probucol on dietary cholesterol-induced atherosclerosis in rabbits. *Free Radic Biol Med* 1998 Jan 15;24(2):226-33.

Preuss HG, Gondal JA, Lieberman S. Association of macroutrients and energy intake with hypertension. *J Am Coll Nutr* 1996; 15(1): 21-35.

Preuss HG, Grojec PL et al. Effects of different chromium compounds on blood pressure and lipid peroxidation in spontaneously hypertensive rats. *Clin Nephrol* 1997; 47(5): 325-30.

Rauchova H, Dobesova Z et al. The effect of chronic L-carnitine treatment on blood pressure and plasma lipids in spontaneously hypertensive rats. *Eur J Pharmacol* 1998; 342(2-3): 235-9.

Simon JA, Hudes ES. Relation of serum ascorbic acid to serum lipids and lipoproteins in US adults. *J Am Coll Nutr* 1998 Jun;17(3):250-5.

Stabler SP, Lindenbaum J, Allen RH. Vitamin B-12 deficiency in the elderly: current dilemmas. *Am J Clin Nutr* 1997; 66(4): 741-9.

Stephens NG, Parsons A et al. Randomised controlled trial of vitamin E in patients with coronary disease: Cambridge Heart Antioxidant Study *Lancet* 1996; 347(9004): 781-6.

Toohey L, Harris MA, et al. Plasma ascorbic acid concentrations are related to cardiovascular risk factors in African-Americans. *J Nutr* 1996 Jan;126(1):121-8.

Van der Griend R, Haas FJ, et al. Combination of low dose folic acid and pyridoxine for treatment of hyperhomocysteinaemia in patients with premature arterial disease and their relatives. *Atherosclerosis* 1999 Mar;143(1):177-83.

Chapter 2 ♡ *Giggling Guts*

Bazhenov LG, Bondarenko VM, et al. The antagonistic action of lactobacilli on Helicobacter pylori. *Zh Mikrobiol Epidemiol Immunobiol* 1997 May-Jun;(3):89-91.

Benno Y, Endo K et al. Comparison of fecal microflora of elderly persons in rural and urban areas of Japan. *Appl Environ Microbiol* 1989; 55(5): 1100-5.

Bjarnason I, MacPherson A, Hollander D. Intestinal permeability: an overview. *Gastroenterology* 1995; 108(5): 1566-81.

Bjarnason I, Hayllar J. Early pathogenic events in NSAID-induced gastrointestinal damage. *Ital J Gastroenterol* 1996; 28 Suppl 4: 19-22.

Bjarnson I, Thjodleifsson B. Gastrointestinal toxicity of non-steriodal anti-inflammatory drugs: the effect of nimesulide compared with naproxen on the human gastrointestinal tract. *Rheumatology (Oxford)* 1999; 38 Suppl 1: 24-32.

Bjorksten B, Naaber P, et al. The intestinal microflora in allergic Estonian and Swedish 2-year-old children. *Clin Exp Allergy* 1999 Mar;29(3):342-6.

Buffington GD, Doe WF. Depleted mucosal antioxidant defenses in inflammatory bowel disease. *Free Rad Biol Med* 1995; 19(6): 911-8.

Buts JP, Bernasconi P, et al. Stimulation of secretory IgA and secretory component of immunoglobulins in small intestine of rats treated with Saccharomyces boulardii. *Dig Dis Sci* 1990 Feb;35(2):251-6.

De Keyser F, Elewaut D et al. Bowel inflammation and the spondyloarthropathies. *Rheum Dis Clin North Am* 1998; 24(4): 785-813.

De Vos M, De Keyser F et al. Review article: bone and joint diseases in inflammatory bowel disease. *Aliment Pharmacol Ther* 1998; 12(5): 397-404.

Elmer GW, Surawicz CM, McFarland LV. Biotherapeutic agents. A neglected modality for the treatment and prevention of selected intestinal and vaginal infections. *JAMA* 1996; 275(11): 870-6.

Fukushima Y, Kawata Y et al. Effect of bifidobacteria feeding on fecal flora and production of immunoglubulins in lactating mouse. *Int J Food Microbiol* 1999; 46(3): 193-7.

Hollander D, Tarnawski A. Is there a role for dietary essential fatty acids in gastroduodenal mucosal protection? *J Clin Gastroenterol* 1991; 13 Suppl 1: S72-4.

Hollander D, Tarnawski H. Aging-associated increase in intestinal absorption of macromolecules. *Gerontology* 1985; 31(3):133-7.

Inman RD. Antigens, the gastrointestinal tract and arthritis. *Rheum Dis Clin No Amer* 1991; 17:309-21.

Jahn HU, Ullrich R, et al. Immunological and trophical effects of Saccharomyces boulardii on the small intestine in healthy human volunteers. *Digestion* 1996; 57(2):95-104.

Kirchhelle A, Fruhwein N, Toburen D. Treatment of persistent diarrhea with S. boulardii in returning travelers. Results of a prospective study. *Fortschr Med* 1996 Apr 20;114(11):136-40.

Litiaeva LA. The effect of a combination of immune and bacterial preparations on the microbial ecology of pregnant women in a risk group. *Akush Ginekol (Mosk)* 1993;(1):19-22.

Lorscheider FL, Vimy MJ et al. The dental amalgam mercury controversy—inorganic mercury and the CNS; genetic linkage of mercury and antibiotic resistances in intestinal bacteria. *Toxicology* 1995; 97(1-3):19-22.

Lykova EA, Bondarenko VM, et al. The probiotic correction of microecological and immune disorders in gastroduodenal pathology in children. *Zh Mikrobiol Epidemiol Immunobiol* 1996 Mar-Apr;(2):88-91.

Ma TY, Hollander D et al. Mechanism of colonic permeation of inulin: is rat colon more permeable than small intestine? *Gastroenterology* 1995; 108(1): 12-20.

Majamaa H, Isolauri E. Probiotics: a novel approach in the management of food allergy. *J Allergy Clin Immunol* 1997; 99(2): 179-85.

Majamaa H, Isolauri E. Evaluation of the gut mucosal barrier: evidence for increased antigen transfer in children with atopic eczema. *J Allergy Clin Immunol* 1996; 97(4): 985-90.

Majumdar AP, Jasewski R, Dubick MA. Effect of aging on the gastrointestinal tract and pancreas. *Proc Soc Exp Biol Med* 1997 Jun;215(2):134-44.

Malin M, Suomalainen H, et al. Promotion of IgA immune response in patients with Crohn's disease by oral bacteriotherapy with Lactobacillus GG. *Ann Nutr Metab* 1996;40(3):137-45.

May T, Mackie RI et al. Effect of fiber source on short-chain fatty acid production and on the growth and toxin production by Clostridium difficile. *Scand J Gastroenterol* 1994; 29(10): 916-22.

McFarland LV. Epidemiology, risk factors and treatments for antibiotic-associated diarrhea. *Dig Dis* 1998; 16(5): 292-307.

McFarland LV et al. Biotherapeutic agents, a neglected modality for the treatment and prevention of selected intestinal and vaginal infections. *JAMA* 1996; 275: 870-6.

McKenzie SJ, Baker MS et al. Evidence of oxidant-induced injury to epithelial cells during inflammatory bowel disease. *J Clin Invest* 1996; 98(1): 136-41.

Mielants H, Veys EM et al. Course of gut inflammation in spondylarthropathies and therapeutic consequences. *Baillieres Clin Rheumatol* 1996; 10(1): 147-64.

Mohan JC, Arora R, Khalilullah M. Short term hypolipidemic effects of oral lactobacillus sporogenes therapy in patients with primary dyslipidemias. *Indian Heart J* 1990 Sep-Oct;42(5):361-4.

Pecorella G, Vasquez E, et al. The effect of Lactobacillus acidophilus and Bifidobacterium bifidum on the intestinal ecosystem of the elderly patient. *Clin Ter* 1992 Jan;140(1):3-10.

Sigthorsson G, Tibble J et al. Intestinal permeability and inflammation in patients on NSAIDS. *Gut* 1998; 43(4): 506-11.

Smith JG, Yokoyama WH, German JB. Butyric acid from the diet: actions at the level of gene expression. *Crit Rev Food Sci Nutr* 1998; 38(4): 259-97.

Swenson ES, Milisen WB, Curatolo W. Intestinal permeability enhancement: Efficacy, acute local toxicity, and reversibility. *Pharmacol Res* 1994; 11(8):1132-42

Tarnawski A, Hollander D, Gergely H. Protection of the gastric mucosa by linoleic acid—a nutrient essential fatty acid. *Clin Invest Med* 1987; 10(3): 132-5.

Tiwana H, Wilson C et al. Antibody responses to gut bacteria in ankylosing spondylitis, rheumatoid arthritis, Crohn's disease and ulcerative colitis. *Rheumatol Int* 1997; 17(1): 11-6.

Wickens K, Pearce N, et al. Antibiotic use in early childhood and the development of asthma. *Clin Exp Allergy* 1999 Jun;29(6):766-71.

Xu X, Harris KS, et al. Bioavailability of soybean isoflavones depends on gut microflora in women. *J Nutr* 1995; 125(9): 2307-15.

Chapter 3 ♡ *Leaping Livers and Nutritional Supplements*

Ames BN, Shigenaga MK, Hagen TM. Oxidants, antioxidants, and the degenerative diseases of aging. *Proc Natl Acad Sci USA* 1993 Sep 1;90(17):7915-22.

Batt AM, Ferrari L. Manifestations of chemically induced liver damage. *Clin Chem* 1995; 41(12 Pt 2):1882-7.

Batt AM, Magdalou J et al. Drug metabolizing enzymes related to laboratory medicine: cytochromes P-450 and UDP-glucuronosyltransferases. *Clin Chim Acta* 1994; 226(2): 171-90.

Batt AM, Siest G et al. Enzyme induction by drugs and toxins. *Clin Chim Acta* 1992; 2029(1-2): 109-21.

Belpaire FM, Bogaert MG. Cytochrome P450: genetic polymorphism and drug interactions. Acta *Clin Belg* 1996; 51(4): 254-60.

Berkson BM. A conservative triple antioxidant approach to the treatment of hepatitis C. Combination of alpha lipoic acid (thioctic acid), silymarin, and selenium: three case histories. *Med Klin* 1999 Oct 15;94 Suppl 3:84-9.

Bradfield CA, Bjeldanes LF. Structure-activity relationships of dietary indoles: a proposed mechanism of action as modifiers of xenobiotic metabolism. *J Toxicol Environ Health* 1987;21(3):311-23.

Brockmoller J, Roots I. Assessment of liver metabolic function. *Clin Pharmicokinet* 1994; 27:216-48.

Cameron NE, Cotter MA, Hohman TC. Interactions between essential fatty acid, prostanoid, polyol pathway and nitric oxide mechanisms in the neurovascular deficit of diabetic rats. *Diabetologia* 1996 Feb;39(2):172-82.

Cameron NE, Cotter MA, et al. Effects of alpha-lipoic acid on neurovascular function in diabetic rats: interaction with essential fatty acids. *Diabetologia* Apr;41(4):390-9.

Carr AC, Frei B. Toward a new recommended dietary allowance for vitamin C based on antioxidant and health effects in humans. *Am J Clin Nutr* 1999 Jun;69(6):1086-107.

Cotter MA, Love A, et al. Effects of natural free radical scavengers on peripheral nerve and neurovascular function in diabetic rats. _Diabetologia_ 1995 Nov;38(11):1285-94.

Cunningham JJ. Micronutrients as nutriceutical interventions in diabetes mellitus. _J Am Coll Nutr_ 1998 Feb;17(1):7-10.

Cunningham JJ, Mearkle PL, Brown RG. Vitamin C: an aldose reductase inhibitor that normalizes erythrocyte sorbitol in insulin-dependent diabetes mellitus. _J Am Coll Nutr_ 1994 Aug;13(4):344-50.

Devlin J, Ellis AE et al. N-acetylcysteine improves indocyanine green extraction and oxygen transport during hepatic dysfunction. _Crit Care Med_ 1997; 25(2): 236-42.

Douillet C, Tabib A, et al. A selenium supplement associated or not with vitamin E delays early renal lesions in experimental diabetes in rats. _Proc Soc Exp Biol Med_ Apr;211(4):323-31.

Forsleff L, Schauss AG, et al. Evidence of functional zinc deficiency in Parkinson's disease. _J Altern Complement Med_ 1999 Feb;5(1):57-54.

Galan P, Preziosi P, et al. Effects of trace element and/or vitamin supplementation on vitamin and mineral status, free radical metabolism and immunological markers in elderly long term-hospitalized subjects. Geriatric Network MIN. VIT. AOX. _Int J Vitam Nutr Res_ 1997;67(6):450-60.

Grimble RF. Effect of antioxidative vitamins on immune function with clinical applications. _Int J Vitam Nutr Res_ 1997;67(5):312-20.

Grimble RF. Nutritional modulation of cytokine biology. _Nutrition_ 1998 Jul-Aug;14(7-8):634-40.

Grimble RF, Grimble GK. Immunonutrition: role of sulfur amino acids, related amino acids, and polyamines. _Nutrition_ 1998 Jul-Aug;14(7-8):605-10.

Hagen TM, Ingersoll RT, et al. Acetyl-L-carnitine fed to old rats partially restores mitochondrial function and ambulatory activity. _Proc Natl Acad Sci USA_ 1998 Aug 4;95(16):9562-6.

Hagen TM, Ingersoll RT, et al. (R)-alpha-lipoic acid-supplemented old rats have improved mitochondrial function, decreased oxidative damage, and increased metabolic rate. _FASEB J_ 1999 Feb;13(2):411-8.

Hemila H, Douglas RM. Vitamin C and acute respiratory infections. _Int J Tuberc Lung Dis_ 1999 Sep;3(9):756-61.

Kagan VE, Shvedova A, et al. Dihydrolipoic acid–a universal antioxidant both in the membrane and in the aqueous phase. Reduction of peroxyl, ascorbyl and chromanoxyl radicals. _Biochem Pharmacol_ 1992 Oct 20;44(8):1637-49.

Keays R, Harrison PM et al. Intravenous acetylcysteine in paracetamol induced fulminant hepatic failure: a prospective controlled trail. _BMJ_ 1991; 303(6809): 1026-9.

Khanna S, Roy S, et al. Cytokine-induced glucose uptake in skeletal muscle: redox regulation and the role of alpha-lipoic acid. _Am J Physiol_ 1999 May;276(5 Pt 2):R1327-33.

Kim H, Wang RS et al. Cytochrome P450 isozymes responsible for the metabolism of toluene and styrene in human liver microsomes. *Xenobiotica* 1997; 27(7): 657-65.

Lykkesfeldt J, Hagen TM, et al. Age-associated decline in ascorbic acid concentration, recycling, and biosynthesis in rat hepatocytes–reversal with (R)-alpha-lipoic acid supplementation. *FASEB J* 1998 Sep;12(12):1183-9.

McCall MR, Frei B. Can antioxidant vitamins materially reduce oxidative damage in humans? *Free Radic Biol Med* 1999 Apr;26(7-8):1034-53.

Medyani M, Lipman RD, et al. The effect of long-term dietary supplementation with antioxidants. *Ann N Y Acad Sci* 1998 Nov 20;854:352-60.

Nappo F, De Rosa N, et al. Impairment of endothelial functions by acute hyperhomocysteinemia and reversal by antioxidant vitamins. *JAMA* 1999 Jun 9;281(22):2113-8.

Naurath HJ, Joosten E, et al. Effects of vitamin B12, folate, and vitamin B6 supplements in elderly people with normal serum vitamin concentrations. *Lancet* 1995 Jul 8;346(8967):85-9.

Nickander KK, McPhee BR, et al. Alpha-lipoic acid: antioxidant potency against lipid peroxidation of neural tissues in vitro and implications for diabetic neuropathy. *Free Radic Biol Med* 1996;21(5):631-9.

Pelkonen O, Raunio H. Metabolic activation of toxins: tissue-specific expression and metabolism in target organs. *Environ Health Perspect* 1997; 105 Suppl 4: 767-74.

Pepersack T, Garbusinski J, et al. Clinical relevance of thiamine status amongst hospitalized elderly patients. *Gerontology* 1999;45(2):96-101.

Savage DG, Lindenbaum J. Neurological complications of acquired cobalamin deficiency: clinical aspects. *Baillieres Clin Haematol* 1995; 8(3): 657-78.

Schiodt FV et al. Acetaminophen toxicity in an urban county hospital. *N Engl J Med* 1997; 337(16):1112-7.

Scott BC, Aruoma OI, et al. Lipoic and dihydrolipoic acids as antioxidants. A critical evaluation. *Free Radic Res* 1994 Feb;20(2):119-33.

Serbinova E, Kagan V, et al. Free radical recycling and intramembrane mobility in the antioxidant properties of alpha-tocopherol and alpha-tocotrienol. *Free Radic Biol Med* 1991;10(5):263-75.

Simon JA, Hudes ES. Serum ascorbic acid and cardiovascular disease prevalence in U.S. adults: the Third National Health and Nutrition Examination Survey (NHANES III). *Ann Epidemiol* 1999 Aug;9(6):358-65.

Simon JA, Hudes ES. Serum ascorbic acid and other correlates of gallbladder disease among US adults. *Am J Public Health* 1998 Aug;88(8):1208-12.

Sotaniemi EA, Arranto AJ et al. Age and cytochrome P450-linked drug metabolism in humans: an analysis of 226 subjects with equal histopathologic conditions. *Clin Pharmacol Ther* 1997; 61(3): 331-9.

Sternberg P Jr, Davidson PC, et al. Protection of retinal pigment epithelium from oxidative injury by glutathione and precursors. *Invest Opthalmol Vis Sci* 1993 Dec;34(13):3661-8.

Tirosh O, Sen CK, et al. Neuroprotective effects of alpha-lipoic acid and its positively charged amide analogue. _Free Radic Biol Med_ 1999 Jun;26(11-12):1418-26.

Traber MG. Cellular and molecular mechanisms of oxidants and antioxidants. _Miner Electrolyte Metab_ 1997;23(3-6):135-9.

Vieth R. Vitamin D supplementation, 25-hydroxyvitamin D concentrations, and safety. _Am J Clin Nutr_ 1999 May;69(5):842-56.

Wallig MA. Xenobiotic metabolism, oxidant stress and chronic pancreatitis. Focus on glutatione. _Digestion_ 1998;59 Suppl 4:13-24.

Wenzel G, Kuklinski B, et al. Alcohol-induced toxic hepatitis–a "free radical" associated disease. Lowering fatality by adjuvant antioxidant therapy. _Z Gesamte Inn Med_ 1993 Oct;48(10):490-6.

Xu DP, Wells WW. alpha-Lipoic acid dependent regeneration of ascorbic acid from dehydroascorbic acid in rat liver mitochondria. _J Bioenerg Biomembr_ 1996 Feb;28(1):77-85.

Chapter 4 ♡ Demystifying Diets

Adlercreutz H. Epidemiology of phyoestrogens. _Bailliers Clin Endocrinol Metab_ 1998 Dec;12(4):605-23.

Adlercreutz H, Mazar W. Phyto-oestrogens and Western diseases. _Ann Med_ 1997 Apr;29(2):95-120.

Appleby PN, Thorogood M, et al. The Oxford Vegetarian Study: an overview. _Am J Clin Nutr_ 1999 Sep;70(3 Suppl):525S-531S.

Beilin LJ. Non-pharmacological management of hypertension: optimal strategies for reducing cardiovascular risk. _J Hypertens Suppl_ 1994 Dec;12(10):S71-81.

Beilin LJ, Burke V. Vegetarian diet components, protein and blood pressure: which nutrients are important? _Clin Exp Pharmacol Physiol_ 1995 Mar;22(3):195-8.

Bourre JM, Durand G, et al. Changes in auditory brainstem responses in alpha-linolenic acid deficiency as a function of age in rats. _Audiology_ 1999 Jan-Feb;38(1):13-8.

Chang-Claude J, Frentzel-Beyme R. Dietary and lifestyle determinants of mortality among German vegetarians. _Int J Epidemiol_ 1993 Apr;22(2):228-36.

Craig WJ. Health-promoting properties of common herbs. _Am J Clin Nutr_ 1999 Sep;70(3 Suppl):491S-499S.

Daniel O, Meier MS, et al. Selected Phenolic Compounds in Cultivated Plants: Ecologic Functions, Health Implications, and Modulation by Pesticides. _Environ Health Perspect_ 1999 Feb;107 Suppl 1:109-114.

Forsythe WA, Green MS, Anderson JJ. Dietary protein effects on cholesterol and lipoprotein concentrations: a review. _J Am Coll Nutr_ 1986;5(6):533-49.

Frentzel-Beyme R, Chang-Claude J. Vegetarian diets and colon cancer: the German experience. _Am J Clin Nutr_ 1994 May;59(5 Suppl):1143S-1152S.

Frost G, Leeds AA, et al. Glycaemic index as a determinant of serum HDL-cholesterol concentration. *Lancet* 1999 Mar 27;353(9158):1045-8.

Hutchins AM, Lampe JW, et al. Vegetables, fruits, and legumes: effect on urinary isoflavanoid phytoestrogen and lignan excretion.*J Am Diet Assoc* 1995 Jul;95(7):769-74.

Kaneyuki T, Noda Y, et al. Superoxide anion and hydroxyl radical scavenging activities of vegetable extracts measured using electron spin resonance.*Biochem Mol Biol Int* 1999 Jun;47(6):979-89.

Key TJ, Fraser Ge, et al. Mortality in vegetarians and nonvegetarians: detailed findings from a collaborative analysis of 5 prospective studies.*Am J Clin Nutr* 1999 Sep;70(3 Suppl):516S-524S.

Keys A. Mediterranean diet and public health: personal reflections. *Am J Clin Nutr* 1995 Jun;61(6 Suppl):1321S-1323S.

Kirkman LM, Lampe JW, et al. Urinary lignan and isoflavanoid excretion in men and women consuming vegetable and soy diets. *Nutr Cancer* 1995;24(1):1-12.

Knight DC, Eden JA. A review of the clinical effects of phytoestrogens.*Obstet Gynecol* 1996; 87(5 Pt 2): 897-904.

Ludwig DS, Majzoub JA, et al. High glycemic index foods, overeating, and obesity. *Pediatrics* 1999 Mar;103(3):E26.

Marcovina SM, Kennedy H, et al. Fish intake, independent of apo(a) size, accounts for lower plasma lipoprotein(a) levels in Bantu fisherman of Tanzania: The Lugalawa Study. *Arterioscler Thromb Vasc Biol* 1999 May;19(5):1250-6.

Mori TA, Vandongen R, et al. Effects of varying dietary fat, fish, and fish oils on blood lipids in a randomized controlled trail in men at risk of heart disease.*Am J Clin Nutr* 1994 May;59(5):1060-8.

Puddey IB, Croft KD, et al. Alcohol, free radicals and antioxidants. *Novartis Found Symp* 1998;216:51-62.

Risch HA, Jain M, et al. Dietary fat intake and risk of epithelial ovarian cancer. *J Natl Cancer Inst* 1994 Sep 21;86(18):1409-15.

Solfrizzi V, Panza F, et al. High monounsaturated fatty acids intake protects against age-related cognitive decline. *Neurology* 1999 May 12;52(8):1563-9.

Vang O, Rasmussen BF, Anderson O. Combined effects of complex mixtures of potentially anti-carcinogenic compounds on antioxidant enzymes and carcinogen metabolizing enzymes in the rat. *Cancer Lett* Mar 19;114(1-2):283-6.

Wiseman H. The bioavailability of non-nutrient plant factors: dietary flavonoids and phyto-oestrogens. *Proc Nutr Soc* 1999 Feb;58(1):139-46.

Wolk A, Manson JE, et al. Long-term intake of dietary fiber and decreased risk of coronary heart disease among women. *JAMA* 1999 Jun 2;281(21):1998-2004.

Yochum L, Kushi LH, et al. Dietary flavonoid intake and risk of cardiovascular disease in postmenopausal women. *Am J Epidemiol* 1999 May 15;149(10):943-9.

Chapter 5 ♡ Glad Glands

Anderson JW, Blake JE et al. Effects of soy protein on renal function and proteinuria in patients with type 2 diabetes. *Am J Clin Nutr* 1998; 68(6 Suppl): 1347S-1353S.

Anderson JW, O'Neal DS et al. Postprandial serum glucose, insulin, and lipoprotein responses to high- and low-fiber diets. *Metabolism* 1995; 44(7): 848-54.

Arjmandi BH, Birnbaum R et al. Bone-sparing effect of soy protein in ovarian hormone-deficient rats is related to its isoflavone content. *Am J Clin Nutr* 1998; 68(6 Suppl): 1364S-1368S.

Arjmandi BH, Getlinger MJ et al. Role of soy protein with normal or reduced isoflavone content in reversing bone loss induced by ovarian hormone deficiency in rats. *Am J Clin Nutr* 1998; 68(6 Suppl): 1358S-1363S.

Barnes S. Phytoestrogens and breast cancer. *Baillieres Clin Metab* 1998; 12(4): 559-79.

Cunningham JJ. The glucose/insulin system and vitamin C: implications in insulin-dependent diabetes mellitus. *J Am Coll Nutr* 1998 Apr;17(2):105-8.

Dou C, Xu DP, Wells WW. Studies on the essential role of ascorbic acid in the energy dependent release of insulin from pancreatic islets. *Biochem Biophys Res Commun* 1997 Feb 24;231(3):820-2.

Estrada DE, Ewart HS, et al. Stimulation of glucose uptake by the natural coenzyme alpha-lipoic acid/thioctic acid: participation of elements of the insulin signaling pathway. *Diabetes* 1996 Dec;45(12):1798-804.

Forsythe WA 3rd. Soy protein, thyroid regulation and cholesterol metabolism. *J Nutr* 1995 Mar;125(3 Suppl):619S-623S.

Fujita T. Clinical guidelines for the treatment of osteoporosis in Japan. *Calcif Tissue Int* 1996; 59 Suppl 1:34-7.

Humphries S, Kushner H, Falkner B. Low dietary magnesium is associated with insulin resistance in a sample of young, nondiabetic Black Americans. *Am J Hypertens* 1999 Aug;12(8 Pt 1):747-56.

Kahler W, Kuklinski B, et al. Diabetes mellitus–a free radical-associated disease. Results of adjuvant antioxidant supplementation. *Z Gesamte Inn Med* 1993 May;48(5):223-32.

Keen H, Payan J, et al. Treatment of diabetic neuropathy with gamma-linoleic acid. The gamma-Linoleic Acid Multicenter Trial Group. *Diabetes Care* 1993 Jan;16(1):8-15.

Kirkman LM, Lampe JW, et al. Urinary lignan and isoflavanoid excretion in men and women consuming vegetable and soy diets. *Nutr Cancer* 1995;24(1):1-12.

Lampe JW, Martini MC, et al. Urinary lignan and isoflavanoid excretion in premenopausal women consuming flaxseed powder. *Am J Clin Nutr* 1994 Jul;60(1):122-8.

Ludwig DS, Pereira MA, et al. Dietary fiber, weight, gain, and cardiovascular disease risk factors in young adults. *JAMA* 1999 Oct 27;282(16):1539-46.

Mori TA, Bao DQ, et al. Dietary fish as a major component of a weight-loss diet: effect on serum lipids, glucose, and insulin metabolism in overweight hypertensive subjects. *Am J Clin Nutr* 1999 Nov;70(5):817-825

Mori TA, Vandongen R, et al. Effects of varying dietary fat, fish, and fish oils on blood lipids in a randomized controlled trail in men at risk of heart disease. *Am J Clin Nutr* 1994 May;59(5):1060-8.

Phipps WR, Martini MC, et al. Effect of flax seed ingestion on the menstrual cycle. *J Clin Endocrinol Metab* 1993 Nov;77(5):1215-9.

Prince R et al. The effects of calcium supplementation (milk powder or tablets) and exercise on bone density in postmenopausal women. *J Bone Miner Res* 1995; 10(7): 1068-75

Ravina A, Slezak L, et al. Reversal of corticosteroid-induced diabetes mellitus with supplemental chromium. *Diabet Med* 1999 Feb;16(2):164-7.

Salmeron J et al. Dietary Fiber, glycemic load, and risk of NIDDM in men. *Diabetes Care* 1997; 20(4):545-50.

Serfaty D, Magneron AC. Premenstrual syndrome in France: epidemiology and therapeutic effectiveness of 1000 mg of micronized purified flavonoid fraction in 1473 gynecological patients. *Contracept Fertil Sex* 1997 Jan;25(1):85-90.

Striffler JS, Polansky MM, Anderson RA. Overproduction of insulin in the chromium-deficient rat. *Metabolism* 1999 Aug;48(8):1063-8.

Tham DM, Gardner CD, Haskell WL. Clinical review 97: Potential health benefits of dietary phyoestrogens: a review of the clinical, epidemiological, and mechanistic evidence. *J Clin Endocrinol Metab* 1998 Jul;83(7):2223-35.

Thomas JA. Diet, micronutrients, and the prostate gland. *Nutr Rev* 1999 Apr;57(4):95-103.

Wang H, Zhang ZB, et al. Experimental and clinical studies on the reduction of erythrocyte sorbitol-glucose ratios by ascorbic acid in diabetes mellitus. *Diabetes Res Clin Pract* 1995 Apr;28(1);1-8.

Wood RJ, Zheng JJ. High dietary calcium intakes reduce zinc absorption and balance in humans. *Am J Clin Nutr* 1997; 65(6): 1803-9.

Wyatt KM, Dimmock PW, et al. Efficacy of vitamin B-6 in the treatment of premenstrual syndrome: systematic review. *BMJ* 1999 May 22;318(7195):1375-81.

Xu X, Duncan AM, et al. Effects of soy isoflavones on estrogen and phytoestrogen metabolism in premenopausal women. *Cancer Epidemiol Biomarkers Prev* 1998 Dec;7(12):1101-8.

Chapter 6 ♡ *Danger Drugs*

Adlerkreutz H, Mazur W. Phyto-oestrogens and Western diseases. *Ann Med* 1997 Apr;29(2):95-120.

Aso Y, Akaza H, et al. Preventive effect of a Lactobacillus casei preparation on the recurrence of superficial bladder cancer in a double-blind trial. The BLP Study Group. *Eur Urol* 1995;27(2):104-9.

Azzi A, Aratri E, et al. Molecular basis of alpha-tocopherol control of smooth muscle proliferation. *Biofactors* 1998;7(1-2):3-14.

Baghurst PA, Tong S et al. Sociodemographic and behavioural determinants of blood lead concentrations in children aged 11-13 years. The Port Pirie Cohort Study. *Med J Aust* 1999; 170(2):63-7.

Bradfield CA, Bjeldanes LF. Modification of carcinogen metabolism by indolylic autolysis products of Brassica oleraceae. *Adv Exp Med Biol* 1991;289:153-63.

Brockmoller J, Cascorbi I et al. Polymorphisms in xenobiotic conjugation and disease predisposition. *Toxicol Lett*; 102-103:173-83.

Burns JM, Baghurst PA et al. Lifetime low-level exposure to environmental lead and children's emotional and behavioral development at ages 11-13 years. The Port Pirie Cohort Study. *Am J Epidemiol* 1999;149(8): 740-9.

Combs GF Jr. Chemopreventive mechanisms of selenium. *Med Klin* 1999 Oct 15;94 Suppl 3:18-24.

Dashwood RH. Early detection and prevention of colorectal cancer (review). *Oncol Rep* 1999 Mar-Apr;6(2):277-81.

el-Fawal HA, Gong Z, et al. Exposure to methylmercury results in serum autoantibodies to neurotypic and gliotypic proteins. *Neurotoxicology* 1996 Spring;17(1):267-76.

Enger SM, Ross RK, et al. Alcohol consumption and breast cancer oestrogen and progesterone receptor status. *Br J Cancer* 1999 Mar;797(7-8):1308-14.

Gong Z, Evans HL. Effect of chelation with meso-dimercaptosuccinic acid (DMSA) before and after the appearance of lead-induced neurotoxicity in the rat. *Toxicol Appl Pharmacol* 1997 Jun;144(2):205-14.

Haggans CJ, Hutchins AM, et al. Effect of flaxseed consumption on urinary estrogen metabolites in postmenopausal women. *Nutr Cancer* 1999;33(2):188-95.

Hu J, La Vecchia C, et al. Diet and brain cancer in adults: a case-control study in northeast China. *Int J Cancer* 1999 Mar 31;81(1):20-3.

Ingram D, Sanders K, et al. Case-control Study of phyto-oestrogens and breast cancer. *Lancet* 1997 Oct 4;350(9083):990-4.

Jacobsen EL, Shieh WM, Huang AC. Mapping the role of NAD metabolism in prevention and treatment of carcinogenesis. *Mol Cell Biochem* 1999 Mar; 193(1-2):69-74.

Jensen TK, Toppari J, et al. Do environmental estrogens contribute to the decline in male reproductive health? *Clin Chem* 1995 Dec;41(12 Pt 2):1896-901.

Levi F, Pasche C, et al. Food groups and colorectal cancer risk. *Br J Cancer* 1999 Mar;79(7-8):1283-7.

Li Y, Upadhyay S, et al. Induction of apoptosis in breast cancer cells MDA-MB-231 by genistein. *Oncogene* 1999 May 20;18(20):3166-72.

Lorscheider FL, Vimy MJ et al. The dental amalgam mercury controversy—inorganic mercury and the CNS; genetic linkage of mercury and antibiotic resistances in intestinal bacteria. *Toxicology* 1995; 97(1-3):19-22.

Lorscheider FL, Vimy MJ, Summers AO. Mercury exposure from "silver" tooth fillings: emerging evidence questions a traditional dental paradigm. *FASEB J* 1995; 9(7): 504-8.

Mottet NK et al. Metabolism of methylmercury in the brain and its toxicological significance. *Met Ions Biol Syst.* 1997; 34: 371-403.

Nebert DW, Ingelman-Sundberg M, Daly AK. Genetic epidemiology of environmental toxicity and cancer susceptibility: human allelic polymorphisms in drug metabolizing enzyme genes, their functional importance and nomenclature issues. *Drug Metab Rev* 1999; 31(2): 467-87.

Nestle M. Broccoli sprouts in cancer prevention. *Nutr Rev* 1998 Apr;56(4 Pt 1):127-30.

Nylander M, Friberg L et al. Mercury accumulation in tissues from dental staff and controls in relation to exposure. *Swed Dent J* 1989; 13(6): 235-43.

Nylander M, Friberg L, Lind B. Mercury concentrations in the human brain and kidneys in relation to exposure from dental amalgam fillings. *Swed Dent J* 1987; 11(5):179-87.

Onat D, Boscoboinik D, et al. Effect of alpha-tocopherol and silibin dihemisuccinate on the proliferation of human skin fibroblasts. *Biotechnol Appl Biochem* 1999 Jun;29 (Pt 3):213-5.

Pastori M, Pfander H, et al. Lycopene in association with alpha-tocopherol inhibits at physiological concentrations proliferation of prostate carcinoma cells. *Biochem Biophys Res Commun* 1998 Sep 29;250(3):582-5.

Pelkonen O, Raunio H. Individual expression of carcinogen-metabolizing enzymes: Cytochrome P4502A. *J Occup Environ Med* 1995; 37: 19-24.

Pendergrass JC et al. Mercury vapor inhalation inhibits binding of GTP to tubulin in rat brain: similarity to a molecular lesion in Alzheimer diseased brain. *Neurotoxicology* 1997; 18(2): 315-24.

Risch HA. Estrogen replacement therapy and risk of epithelial ovarian cancer. *Gynecol Oncol* 1996 Nov;63(2):254-7.

Risch HA, Jain M, et al. Dietary fat intake and risk of epithelial ovarian cancer. *J Natl Cancer Inst* 1994 Sep 21;86(18):1409-15.

Schiodt FV et al. Acetaminophen toxicity in an urban county hospital. *N Engl J Med* 1997; 337(16):1112-7.

Shertzer HG, Nebert DW et al. Dioxin causes a sustained oxidative stress response in the mouse. *Biochem Biophys Res Commun* 1998; 253(1): 44-8.

Simon JA, Hudes ES. Relationship of ascorbic acid to blood lead levels. *JAMA* 1999 Jun 23-30;281(24):2289-93.

Staessen JA, Roels HA, et al. Environmental exposure to cadmium, forearm bone density, and risk of fractures: prospective population study. Public Health and

Environmental Exposure to Cadmium (PheeCad) Study Group. *Lancet* 1999 Apr 3;353(9159):1140-4.

Tong S, Baghurst PA et al. Declining blood lead levels and changes in cognitive function during childhood: the Port Pirie Cohort Study. *JAMA* 1998; 280(22): 1915-9.

Wickens K, Pearce N, et al. Antibiotic use in early childhood and the development of asthma. *Clin Exp Allergy* 1999 Jun;29(6):766-71.

Witsell DL, Garrett CG, et al. Effect of Lactobacillus acidophilus on antibiotic-associated gastrointestinal morbidity: a prospective randomized trial. *J Otolaryngol* 1995 Aug;24(4):230-3.

Wossmann W, Kohl M, et al. Mercury intoxication presenting with hypertension and tachycardia. *Arch Dis Child* 1999 Jun;80(6):556-7.

Xu M, Dashwood RH. Chemoprevention studies of heterocyclic amine-induced colon carcinogenesis. *Cancer Lett* 1999 Sep 1;143(2):179-83.

Sources and Resources

Bland, Ph.D., Jeffrey, and Benum, M.A., Sara. *The 20-Day Rejuvenation Diet Program: With the Revolutionary Phytonutrient Diet.* New Canaan, Connecticut: Keats Publishing, Inc., 1997.

Casdorph, Dr. H. Richard, and Walker, Dr. Morton. *Toxic Metal Syndrome: How Metal Poisonings Can Affect Your Brain.* Garden City Park, New York: Avery Publishing Group, 1995.

Castleman, Michael. *The Healing Herbs.* Emmaus, Pennsylvania: Rodale Press, 1991.

Chaitow, Leon. *Vaccination and Immunization: Dangers, Delusions and Alternatives.* Essex, England: The C.W. Daniel Company Limited, 1987.

Colbin, Annemarie. *The Book of Whole Meals.* New York, New York: Ballantine Books, 1983.

Colbin, Annemarie. *Food and Healing.* New York, New York: Bantam Books, 1986.

Crook, M.D., William G. *The Yeast Connection: A Medical Breakthrough.* New York, New York: Random House, 1986.

D'Adamo, Peter, and Whitney, Catherine. *Eat Right for Your Type: The Individualized Diet Solution to Staying Healthy, Living Longer & Achieving Your Ideal Weight.* New York, New York: G.P. Putnam's Sons, 1996.

Diamond, Harvey, and Diamond, Marilyn. *Fit for Life.* New York, New York: Warner Books, 1985.

Eades, M.D., Michael, and Eades, M.D., Mary Dan. *Protein Power.* New York, New York: Bantam Books, 1998.

Erasmus, Udo. *Fats that Heal Fats that Kill.* Burnaby, BC, Canada: Alive Books, 1993.

Erdmann, Ph.D., Robert, and Jones, Meirion. *The Amino Revolution.* New York, New York: Fireside, 1987.

Gotschall, B.A., M.Sc., Elaine. *Breaking the Viscious Cycle: Intestinal Health Through Diet.* Baltimore, Ontario, Canada: The Kirkton Press, 1998.

Hagler, Louise, and Bates, Dorothy, Eds. *The New Farm Vegetarian Cookbook.* Summertown, Tennessee: The Book Publishing Company.

Hardy, Dr. James E. *Mercury Free: The wisdom behind the global consumer movement to ban "silver" dental fillings.* Gabriel Rose Press, Inc., 1996.

Hoffmann, David. *The Holistic Herbal.* The Park Forres, Scotland: The Findhorn Press, 1986.

Hunter, Linda Mason. *The Healthy Home: An Attic-to-Basement Guide to Toxin-Free Living.* Emmaus, Pennsylvania: Rodale Press, 1989.

Kaiser, M.D., Jon D. *Immune Power.* New York, New York: St. Martin's Press, 1993.

Kushi, Michio. *The Macrobiotic Way: The Complete Macrobiotic Diet and Exercise Book.* Garden City Park, New York: Avery Publishing Group Inc., 1993.

Lappé, Francis Moore. *Diet for a Small Planet.* New York, New York: Ballantine Books, 1982.

Lappé, Marc. *When Antibiotics Fail: Restoring the Ecology of the Body.* Berkeley, California: North Atlantic Books, 1986.

McDougall, M.D., John A. *The McDougall Program: Twelve Days to Dynamic Health.* New York, New York: Plume, 1990.

Moyers, Bill. *Healing and the Mind.* New York, New York: Doubleday, 1993.

Murray, N.D., Michael T. *Natural Alternatives to Over-the-Counter and Prescription Drugs.* New York, New York: William Morrow and Company, Inc., 1994.

Murray, N.D., Michael, and Pizzorno, N.D., Joseph. *Encyclopedia of Natural Medicine.* Rocklin, California: Prima Publishing, 1991.

Panos, M.D., Maesimund, and Heimlich, Jane. *Homeopathic Medicine at Home: Natural Remedies for Everday Ailments and Minor Injuries.* Los Angeles, California: J. P. Tarcher, Inc., 1980.

Pelton, R.Ph., Ph.D., Ross, and Overholser, Ph.D., Lee. *Alternatives in Cancer Therapy: The Complete Guide to Non-Traditional Treatments.* New York, New York: Fireside, 1994.

Quillin, Ph.D., R.D., Patrick, and Quillin, Noreen. *Beating Cancer with Nutrition.* Tulsa, Oklahoma: The Nutrition Times Press, Inc., 1994.

Riggs, Maribeth. *Natural Child Care: A Complete Guide to Safe and Effective Herbal Remedies and Holistic Health Strategies for Infants and Children.* New York, New York: Harmony Books, 1989.

Rockwell, Sally J. *Sally Rockwell's Allergy Recipes.* Seattle, Washington: Nutrition Survival Press, 1987.

Shurtleff, William, and Aoyagi, Akiko. *The Book of Tofu: Food for Mankind.* New York, New York: Ballantine Books, 1979.

Weed, Susun S. *Wise Woman Herbal: Healing Wise.* Woodstock, New York: Ash Tree Publishing, 1989.

Weil, M.D., Andrew. *Spontaneous Healing.* New York, New York: Ballantine Books, 1995.

Werbach, M.D., Melvyn. *Healing With Food.* New York, NewYork: Harper Collins, 1993.

Whitaker, M.D., Julian M. *Reversing Diabetes.* New York, New York: Warner Books, 1987.

Index

acetaminophen 65
acidophilus 52-54, 169, 182, 192
adrenal 3, 58, 62, 117, 118, 123-129, 134, 135, 139, 163, 169-171, 174
adrenalin 118, 124-126, 169
airborne allergies 120
alanine 142, 169
albumin 57, 169
alcoholism 29, 39, 136, 169
aldosterone 124, 126-129, 169
allergic reactions 13, 14, 16, 24, 39, 40, 52, 73, 171
aluminum 3, 64, 84, 85, 114, 115, 143, 147, 150, 151, 153, 154
Alzheimer's disease 151, 169
amino acids 2, 40, 78, 79, 119, 127, 138, 139, 142, 159, 169, 184
amylase 30, 50, 169
androgens 124, 126, 129, 169
anise 50
antibiotic 36-38, 41, 52, 113, 114, 161, 169, 182, 183, 191, 192
antibiotics 37, 38, 43, 64, 72, 92, 113, 161, 162, 167, 178, 194
antibodies 35, 40-43, 104, 151, 161, 169
Anti-Candida Diet 97
anti-inflammatories 80
anti-inflammatory 16, 23, 169, 181
anti-microbial 169
anti-oxidants 13, 169
anxiety 131
apples 17, 72, 76, 113
arsenic 3, 92, 112, 143, 150, 153
artificial colors 73
asthma vi, 29, 38, 39, 42, 120, 127, 169, 183, 192, 203
atherosclerosis 3-6, 8, 13, 19, 20, 23, 25, 88, 169, 180
B vitamins 18, 25, 31, 32, 49, 55, 64, 74, 79, 80, 85, 86, 100, 136, 141
B12 25, 31, 49, 139, 141, 185
bacteria 18, 36-39, 41, 46, 52-54, 63, 64, 81, 94, 112, 137, 161, 169, 171, 174, 176, 182, 183, 191
bad cholesterol 8, 9, 13, 24, 25, 58, 121
bad fats 10, 12, 13, 64, 72, 136, 138, 159, 178
beans 17, 19, 46, 47, 72, 93-95, 98, 101, 104-107, 109, 113, 114
beef 15, 16, 64, 106, 107, 113, 114, 148
beneficial bacteria 39, 52, 94, 161, 169, 176
benign prostatic hypertrophy 117, 135, 137
bifidobacter 52, 54, 169
bile 33, 34, 37, 48, 50, 59, 82, 163, 169, 171, 172
bitter herbs 50
black cohosh 132, 140, 141
black currant oil 11, 24, 53, 80
black currant seed oil 136
bleach 71, 72, 146
bloating 44, 54, 130, 132, 177
blood type A 105, 107
blood type AB 105, 107
blood type B 105-107
blood type diets 2, 104, 107, 111
blood type O 105, 107
blood vessels 2, 6, 8, 9, 18, 20, 25, 54, 89, 125, 128, 158
blue-green algae 84
bone loss 140, 141, 188
bone mineral density 130, 141
borage oil 24, 53, 136
boron 79, 141, 160
bowel 17, 18, 29, 36-39, 42, 46, 48, 52, 91, 130, 181, 182
breasts 130
broccoli 7, 8, 75, 76, 104, 109, 149, 155, 160, 191
bromelain 23, 24, 50, 169
Brussels sprouts 7, 75, 109, 149, 160
butter vi, 8, 13-15, 104, 114
B-complex 85, 139
cabbage 7, 74, 75, 78, 95, 109, 149,

155, 160
cabbage family 74, 75, 78, 95
cadmium 3, 84, 112, 143, 150, 151, 154, 191, 192
caffeine 61, 64, 65, 82, 108, 141
calcium 2, 4, 49, 75, 76, 79, 82, 83, 85, 86, 113, 120, 125-128, 136, 139-141, 150, 160, 166, 189
calcium carbonate 82, 83, 141
calcium citrate 85, 141
cancer vi, 3, 4, 48, 67, 73, 82, 94, 142-145, 156-160, 165, 186-192, 194
cancer prevention 3, 143, 156, 157, 159, 191
Candida 3, 29, 38, 39, 41, 43, 46, 54, 97-99, 111, 161, 162, 169, 170, 177
candidiasis 43, 170
carbohydrate 16, 78, 98, 103, 104, 111, 172, 179
carbohydrate block 103
carnitine 26, 170, 180, 184
carotenoids 7, 24, 75, 170
carpet 147, 154
cataracts 128
cauliflower 7, 75, 109, 149, 155, 160
cell receptors 137, 170
cellulase 50, 170
charbroiling 73
chasteberry 140, 170
chelation 155, 156, 170, 190
chemical additives 73
chemicals 14, 15, 34, 64-70, 73, 84, 97, 112-114, 118, 143-149, 157-159, 166, 167, 176
chlorine 72, 112
chromium 55, 79, 85, 121, 136, 138, 139, 160, 180, 189
chronic fatigue 29, 39, 43, 66, 68, 71, 144, 161, 170, 203
chronic fatigue syndrome 29, 66, 68, 71, 144, 161, 170, 203
cigarette 141, 154, 158
cilantro 50

citrus 76, 109, 115, 153
coffee 11, 48, 51, 82, 96, 97, 105-107, 140, 154
colitis vi, 42, 51, 54, 170, 183
colloidal minerals 84
colon 3, 17, 18, 35-37, 41, 45, 46, 52, 54, 69, 82, 100, 137, 157, 161, 167, 169, 170, 176, 182, 186, 192
congestive heart failure 4, 170
constipation 45, 47, 48, 52, 163, 166
CoQ-10 25, 26, 170
corticosteroids 38, 65, 118, 120, 123, 162, 170
cortisol 124, 126-129, 170, 174, 178
cottonseed oil 14, 115
cumin 50
cysteine 78, 79, 170
dairy 15, 16, 42, 72, 73, 75-77, 84, 91, 92, 94, 95, 99, 100, 105-107, 113, 114
dandelion 50, 95
deep frying 73, 158
dehydration 128
delayed food allergies 39, 170
depression 67, 127, 131, 133, 152, 164, 170
dermatitis 29, 38, 39, 170
detoxification 2, 3, 7, 55, 59, 60, 62, 68, 71, 108, 112, 145, 153, 155-157, 170, 177
Detoxification Diet 108, 112
DHEA 118, 129, 170
diabetes vi, 22, 42, 57, 68, 89, 104, 111, 123, 124, 138, 162, 164, 170, 178, 184, 188, 189, 195, 203
diarrhea 48, 49, 52, 114, 163, 181, 182
diets 2, 3, 9-11, 16, 17, 63, 87-90, 93, 95, 97, 99, 100, 104, 105, 107, 108, 110, 111, 114, 123, 176, 177, 186-188
digestion 30-36, 41, 44, 49, 50, 55, 76, 91, 92, 113, 120, 122, 125, 169, 173, 181, 186
digestive enzymes 23, 32, 49, 50, 91, 120, 170

digestive tract 29, 30, 35, 39-41, 44, 45, 49, 50, 54, 58, 105, 108, 157, 167, 171
dioxin 68, 191
diuretics 128, 165, 171
dizziness 43, 164, 166
dong quai 132, 140
dopamine 124, 125, 153, 171, 178
eggs vi, 42, 92, 95, 98-100, 108, 114, 173
endocrine glands 21, 62, 117, 118, 135, 136, 138, 171
enzymes 20, 23, 24, 32-34, 41, 44, 45, 49, 50, 60, 61, 76, 91, 120, 142, 145, 157, 162, 163, 170, 171, 173, 177, 183, 187, 191
ephedra 126, 139, 171
epinephrine 124-126, 171
essential fatty acids vii, 2-4, 10, 11, 15, 16, 24, 47, 51-53, 80, 103, 111, 132, 136, 140, 142, 159, 173, 176, 178, 181, 183
estradiol 134, 165, 171
estrogen 58, 90, 118, 129-134, 136, 137, 140, 141, 145, 165, 171, 174, 189-191
estrogenic herbs 140, 171
evening primrose oil 11, 24, 53, 80
exercise 2, 20, 25, 68, 89, 100, 124, 140, 141, 189, 194
fat vi, 2, 4, 6-10, 12-17, 19, 21, 23, 34, 45, 46, 50, 59, 62, 68, 88-90, 94, 100-104, 110, 111, 113, 121, 122, 127, 130, 136, 145, 159, 162, 163, 169, 172, 173, 175, 176, 180, 187, 189, 191
fiber vii, 17-19, 45-48, 50, 52, 54, 76, 77, 94, 109, 171, 176, 182, 187-189
fibromyalgia 49, 66, 68, 71, 144, 145, 161, 171, 203
fish 10, 15, 16, 24, 47, 53, 74, 77, 80, 93, 94, 98-100, 103-106, 110, 114, 136, 167, 180, 187, 189
fish oil 24, 53
Fit for Life 90-92, 96, 99, 107, 111, 193

flax seed 51, 137, 189
folic acid 25, 49, 141, 171, 180
food combining 91
food sensitivities 29, 38, 39, 41, 42, 48, 52, 108, 203
FOS 54, 171
free range 15
fruit 46, 76, 77, 91-93, 96-98, 104, 106, 107, 109, 110, 115, 147
fungi 37, 38, 97, 161, 171
fungicides 154, 171
gall bladder 33, 34, 37, 59, 137, 164, 169, 171
garden chemicals 65, 143, 146, 147, 166
garlic 17, 21-23, 109, 149, 160
gastrointestinal system 29, 138, 171
GI tract 33, 35, 38, 41, 42, 44, 46, 47, 51, 55, 58, 157, 171
ginger 50, 96
Gingko 26, 54, 78
globulin 57, 171
glucagon 102, 118, 120-123, 126, 138, 171, 178
glues 143, 147
glutamine 51, 53, 54, 81, 119, 138, 142, 171, 172
glutathione 78, 160, 171, 185
glycemic index 102, 103, 109, 110, 171, 187
glycine 142, 172
glycogen 45, 121, 122, 125, 127, 172
good cholesterol 8, 13, 21, 23, 58, 130, 176
gout 22, 172
grapefruit 76
grass fed 15
gut vii, 3, 29, 35-44, 47, 53, 54, 58, 63, 68, 91, 102, 125, 137, 141, 157, 163, 167, 171, 172, 174, 182, 183
H2 blockers 65, 172
hardening of the arteries 4, 10, 13, 27, 169

hawthorne 26
HDL 8, 13, 14, 21-23, 58, 130, 172, 176, 187
headache 66, 67, 166
heart vi, vii, 2-8, 10, 14, 16-20, 25-27, 88, 89, 100, 104, 111, 123, 125, 133, 134, 152, 158, 165, 166, 170, 171, 179, 180, 182, 187, 189
heart attacks 4, 5, 8, 89, 100, 171
heart disease vi, 3, 4, 6, 10, 14, 17, 19, 20, 25, 27, 88, 89, 104, 111, 123, 133, 187, 189
heart rhythm 5, 171
heavy metals 3, 69, 112, 148, 150-152, 155, 157, 178
hepatitis 63, 68, 172, 183
herbicides 14, 64, 65, 72, 143, 145, 148, 158, 167, 178
high blood pressure vi, 89, 100, 104, 123, 151, 152, 162, 166
homocysteine 25, 172
hormone 36, 39, 46, 52, 58, 71, 72, 102, 103, 114, 118-120, 122, 123, 125, 127, 128, 130-132, 135-138, 140, 160, 163, 164, 169-172, 174, 175, 188
household cleaners 72
hydrochloric acid 49, 172
hydrogenated fats 12-14, 136, 176, 180
hydrogenated oils 14, 15, 72, 113, 115, 167
hypoallergenic diet 47, 172
hypoglycemia 111, 124, 125, 172
immune system 16, 24, 35, 37-42, 46, 53, 57-59, 71, 99, 119, 120, 128, 145, 151, 152, 156, 158, 169, 170
indigestion 42, 44, 54, 65, 97
infection 38, 43, 63, 161
inflammatory arthritis 29, 39
insomnia 133
insulin 94, 102, 103, 118, 120-124, 126, 127, 130, 138, 139, 172, 177, 178, 184, 188, 189
insulin resistance 123, 124, 172, 188

insulin shock 124
intestinal lining 41, 51, 53, 54, 81, 117, 172
intestinal permeability 3, 29, 38, 39, 41, 42, 172, 181-183
intestines 3, 17, 31-35, 40, 41, 43, 46, 51, 58, 59, 63, 81, 91, 94, 125, 130, 161, 163, 167, 171, 173
iodine 79, 119, 138
iron 13, 49, 74, 79, 80, 136, 150
irritability 127, 131, 152
irritable bowel syndrome 42
junk food 20, 44
kale 7, 75, 76, 149, 160
kidneys 43, 47, 59, 64, 76, 77, 88, 102, 111, 117, 124, 128, 140, 151, 152, 166, 171, 191
large intestine 35, 36, 40, 45, 46, 48, 51, 53, 54, 63, 70, 81, 82, 94, 137, 161, 163, 170
laxatives 128
LDL 8, 9, 13, 14, 24, 58, 172, 176
lead 3, 70, 83-85, 143, 150-152, 154, 166, 190-192
leaky gut syndrome 3, 29, 172
licorice 50, 128, 132, 139, 140
lipase 50, 172
lipoic acid 24, 25, 78, 80, 139, 149, 155, 159, 172, 183-186, 188
lithium 138, 139, 172
liver detox pathway 61, 64, 172
low fat diets 176
low-calorie diets 63, 88, 89
lymphatic system 43, 172
l-glutamine 81, 172
macrobiotic diet 93-97, 99, 111, 194
magnesium 18, 49, 55, 64, 79, 82, 85, 125, 128, 136, 139, 141, 160, 165, 180, 188
mal-absorption 173
manganese 79, 141, 150, 153, 160, 178
manic depression 67
manufactured home 146

margarine vi, vii, 12-15, 72, 96, 158, 176
maritime pine 54
McDougall 100, 101, 107, 111, 194
menopause 58, 67, 90, 133, 134
menstrual cycle 131, 189
mercury 3, 69, 70, 79, 143, 150-156, 182, 191, 192, 194
methionine 25, 78, 79, 160, 173
milk thistle 78, 149, 155, 173
mitochondria 25, 26, 66, 173, 186
mold 97, 98
monounsaturated 10, 12, 13, 103, 173, 187
MSM 160, 173
mucosa 36-38, 51, 173, 183
mucosal lining 18, 34-36, 41, 42, 51, 133, 173
multiple sclerosis 67, 70, 144, 152, 173, 203
muscle wasting 127, 162
Natural Hygiene 90
neurotoxin 70, 152, 173
niacin 21-23, 173, 179, 180
nightshade family 95, 173
nutrasweet 82, 113, 115
nutritional yeast 100
oils 8, 10-16, 72, 80, 94, 98, 100, 101, 103, 113, 115, 136, 157, 158, 167, 176, 180, 187, 189
olive oil 10, 11, 103, 104, 110, 114
omega 3 10, 11, 16, 24, 103, 173, 176
omega 6 24, 103, 173
onion 75, 78
onions 7, 17, 95, 96, 109, 149, 160
organically grown 72, 76, 93, 113, 114, 149
organophosphate compounds 65, 173
osteoporosis 89, 90, 113, 117, 127-129, 133, 134, 140, 141, 151, 162, 173, 188
ovaries 117, 118, 129, 140, 173
oxidation 11, 13, 24, 25, 173, 176
P450 enzymes 60, 173, 177

paints 143, 147, 154
pancreas 32, 34, 49, 117, 118, 120-124, 138, 139, 169, 171-173, 177, 182
pancreatic enzymes 32-34, 41, 45, 173
pantethine 23, 174
Parkinson's Disease 67, 153, 174, 184
pasta 19, 20, 43, 47, 77, 91, 95, 104, 105, 110
peanut 14, 40
pepsin 31, 41, 45, 49, 174
perfume 66, 67
pesticides 14, 64, 65, 72, 143, 145, 148, 149, 154, 158, 167, 178, 186
phosphatides 81
phosphatidyl choline 81, 174
phosphatidyl inositol 81, 174
phosphorus 82, 83, 113, 128
phytonutrients 7, 46, 47, 74-76, 137, 159
phytosterols 75, 142, 174, 178
pineapple 23, 24, 50, 76, 169
pituitary 117, 118, 140, 174
plaquing 20, 23
plastics 143, 145, 154
PMS 3, 67, 131, 132, 136, 137, 140
pollution 3
polyunsaturated 10, 12, 13, 136, 157, 158, 167
pork 15, 106, 107, 148
potassium 83, 126, 128, 165, 166
poultry 15, 16, 47, 64, 72, 73, 77, 94, 98-100, 104, 105, 110, 113, 114, 149
prednisone 38, 65, 120, 123, 127, 128, 161, 162, 174
premarin 160, 164, 174
prescription drugs 2, 21, 64, 128, 160, 165, 194
preservatives 64, 73, 108, 113, 147, 158, 178
proanthocyanadin 76, 174
probiotics 52, 54, 174, 182
progesterogenic herbs 140, 174
progesterone 58, 118, 123, 126,

129-134, 137, 140-142, 165, 174, 190
prostaglandins 34, 129, 133, 174
prostate 3, 134, 135, 142, 174, 189, 191
protease 24, 50, 174
protein block 103
protein digestion 32, 41, 44
prozac 160, 163, 164
pycnogenol 26, 54, 74, 76, 78, 174
quercitin 54, 174
quinoa 77, 105, 106, 108, 174
rancid oils 72
refined sugars 18, 19, 64, 73, 82, 94, 98
refined sweets 123
relaxin 129, 174
rotation diet 99
salad dressing 7, 8, 101
saliva 31, 34, 44, 45, 169, 174
saw palmetto 142
sea vegetables 93-95
seizure disorders 67
selenium 24, 25, 55, 79, 136, 149, 150, 159, 174, 183, 184, 190
sewage sludge 112, 155
soda 48, 106, 107, 121, 123, 153
sodium 83, 109, 126, 128, 130, 141
soluble fiber 17, 47, 52, 76
solvents 143, 147
somatostatin 122, 123, 174
soy 17, 46, 47, 74, 75, 77, 81, 84, 93-96, 98-101, 107, 109, 110, 113, 132, 136, 137, 140-142, 158, 174, 178, 179, 187-189
soy isoflavones 136, 137, 140-142, 174, 178, 189
spinal cord disease 70
spleen 43, 162
squashes 7, 75, 95, 101, 149
starvation 63, 88
stomach 31-35, 40, 41, 44, 45, 49, 50, 55, 78, 80, 83, 91, 92, 102, 105, 117, 122, 130, 163, 164, 171, 172, 174
stomach acid 31, 32, 34, 41, 44, 45, 49, 50, 55, 105

stroke vi, 3, 4, 6, 8, 13, 123, 130, 164, 165, 180
sulphur 75, 78, 79, 101, 109, 149, 159
Syndrome X 122, 123
tagamet 65, 166, 177
taurine 26, 78, 79, 155, 160, 174
tempeh 47, 74, 75, 93-95, 132, 137, 140, 141, 174, 178
testicles 117, 118, 129, 134, 135
testosterone 58, 118, 129, 130, 134-137, 174
thyroglobulin 119, 175
thyroid 3, 58, 62, 117-120, 138, 163, 175, 188
thyroxine 119, 120, 123, 138, 175
tofu 47, 74-77, 93, 95, 104, 109, 115, 132, 137, 140-142, 175, 178, 195
toxic chemicals 14, 66-68, 70, 84, 113, 114, 143-146, 148, 149, 157, 159
toxic metals 69, 84, 85, 112, 143, 147, 150, 152, 154-157, 167
toxic residues 113
toxins 7, 37, 38, 59, 63-65, 68, 71, 91, 108, 112, 113, 143, 144, 159, 170, 172, 178, 183, 185
triglycerides 21, 23, 58, 100, 121-123, 145, 165, 166, 175
Tums 83
tyrosine 119, 125, 138, 175
urethra 133, 135, 174, 175
urine 76, 88, 128, 140, 174, 175
uterus 130, 131, 175
vagina 130, 133, 134
vegan diet 99, 101
vegetarian 93, 99, 100, 105, 107, 186, 193
viruses 64, 169, 175
vitamin B5 23, 174
vitamin B6 25, 174, 185
vitamin C 24, 49, 55, 78, 80, 84, 109, 134, 136, 139, 149, 159, 180, 183, 184, 188
vitamin D 141, 186

vitamin E 24, 26, 55, 78, 80, 85, 94, 136, 139, 149, 159, 179, 180, 184
vitex 140
water retention 130
weight gain 68, 89, 127, 132
weight loss 68, 87-89, 126
wheat 17-19, 42, 43, 46, 47, 72-74, 77, 84, 93, 96, 98, 99, 105-108, 113, 115
wheat bran 17, 18
white flour 18, 19, 73, 95, 123, 167
white sugar 18

whole grains 11, 17, 19, 46, 47, 74, 77, 93, 94, 97, 98, 100, 101, 111
wild yam 132, 140, 141
yeast 3, 29, 37, 39, 43, 63, 84, 95, 97, 98, 100, 161, 162, 169, 193
yeast infection 43, 63
zinc 49, 55, 79, 85, 134, 139, 141, 142, 160, 179, 184, 189
Zone Diet 2, 101-104, 107, 111

About the Author:

Usha Honeyman, D.C., DABCI is a chiropractic internist, natural health physician, and nutritional counselor. She has a Bachelor of Science degree in human biology, four years of college to become a chiropractic physician, and is a Diplomate of the American Board of Chiropractic Internists. She also has post graduate training at the National College of Naturopathic Medicine (specializing in nutrition and herbs), and twelve years in private practice. She specializes in treating people who have serious illnesses with natural treatments, not drugs.

Dr. Usha Honeyman treats diseases (like arthritis, asthma, chronic fatigue syndrome, diabetes, fibromyalgia, and multiple sclerosis) with nutritional supplements and diet. She provides her patients with detailed evaluation of metabolism using laboratory blood tests to find nutritional imbalances, food sensitivities, and functional problems. She believes everyone has the right to feel vibrantly healthy and that good, balanced information on this topic is unavailable to the public in our current health care system. Whether one feels well, under the weather, or has a serious disease we all have the right to information that will help us feel better and stay healthier over the long term. She routinely spends 45 minutes with each patient because of her strong belief in her responsibility to teach why and how to make lifestyle changes that will alleviate or eliminate health problems.